Breast Cancer in Nigeria: Diagnosis, Management and Challenges

Erhabor Osaro

authorHOUSE®

AuthorHouse™ UK
1663 Liberty Drive
Bloomington, IN 47403 USA
www.authorhouse.co.uk
Phone: 0800.197.4150

© 2016 Erhabor Osaro. All rights reserved.

No part of this book may be reproduced, stored in a retrieval system, or transmitted by any means without the written permission of the author.

Published by AuthorHouse 03/08/2016

ISBN: 978-1-5049-9676-1 (sc)
ISBN: 978-1-5049-9675-4 (hc)
ISBN: 978-1-5049-9677-8 (e)

Print information available on the last page.

Any people depicted in stock imagery provided by Thinkstock are models, and such images are being used for illustrative purposes only. Certain stock imagery © Thinkstock.

This book is printed on acid-free paper.

Because of the dynamic nature of the Internet, any web addresses or links contained in this book may have changed since publication and may no longer be valid. The views expressed in this work are solely those of the author and do not necessarily reflect the views of the publisher, and the publisher hereby disclaims any responsibility for them.

Breast Cancer in Nigeria: Diagnosis, Management and Challenges

Erhabor O [1], Abdulrahaman Y[1], Retsky M [2], Forget P [3], Vaidya Jayant [4], Bello O [5], Adias TC [6], Dagana A [7], Egenti BN [8], Mainasara AS [9], Sahabi SM [10], Rilwanu TI [10], Ahmed Y [11], Hassan M [11], Ajayi O. Ifedayo [12], Okara GC [13,] Lori J [14], Ibiang L [15].

Department of Haematology Faculty of Medical Laboratory Science Usmanu Danfodiyo University, Sokoto, Nigeria [1], Harvard TH Chan School of Public Health Boston MA USA [2], Department of Anesthesiology, Universite catholique de Louvain, St-Luc Hospital, Av. Hippocrate 10-1821, 1200 Brussels, Belgium [3], University College Hospital, London [4], Faculty of Basic Medical Sciences Usmanu Danfodiyo University Sokoto [5], Medical Laboratory Science Department Niger Delta University Amassoma Bayelsa State [6], Department of Haematology University of Abuja Teaching Hospital Teaching Hospital [7], Department of Community Medicine University of Abuja, Nigeria [8], Department of Clinical Biochemistry Faculty of Medical Laboratory Science Usmanu Danfodiyo University, Sokoto, Nigeria [9], Department of Histopathology Usmanu Danfodiyo University Teaching Hospital Sokoto, Nigeria [10], Department of Obstetrics and Gynaecology Usmanu Danfodiyo University Teaching Hospital Sokoto, Nigeria [11], Department of Physiology University of Benin [12], Dr. Hassan's Hospital & Diagnostic Centre, Abuja, Nigeria [13], Bingham University Karu, Abuja, Nigeria [14], Management Sciences for Health (MSH) Abuja, Nigeria [15].

Preface

Worldwide, breast cancer is the commonest cancer in women and it is characterized by regional variations and late clinical presentation and poor access in low and middle income countries including Nigeria. It is disproportionately responsible for mortality among women in developing countries compared to those in developed countries. There are several challenges associated with the effective management of breast cancer in Nigeria; financial barriers limit women's access to screening and treatment services, late-stage presentation, high incidence of triple negative breast cancers and failure in stewardship by government in their inability to provide the best possible cancer care as their counterparts in the West. There is an urgent need to step up activities through governmental and non-governmental agencies to promote advocacy, national policy on training of personnel for diagnosis, clinical and self-breast examination and nationwide screening program (mammography) in order to enhance early detection, control the upward trends and reduce the mortality rate of breast cancer. Routine age appropriate and specific breast screening should become an integral part of healthcare system in Nigeria allowing for early detection and intervention; aggressive awareness campaign on the advantages of early diagnosis and the dangers of late presentation, need to offer universal and affordable treatment, implementation of a strategy to offer annual mammogram to women above the age threshold for breast cancer, increased budgetary allocation for the diagnosis and management of cancer, more investment in the training of healthcare workers involved in the diagnosis and management of breast cancer, provision of health education encouraging women to conduct routine Breast Self Examination (BSE). BSE could become a simple, low-priced, secure, effective, appropriate and feasible screening tool in Nigeria. There is need to re-emphasize the importance of prompt reporting of any new breast symptoms to a health professional. Clinical Breast Examination (CBE) should become part of a periodic health examination, preferably at least every three years. Asymptomatic women aged 40 and over should be offered a CBE as part of a periodic health examination, preferably annually. Objective implementation of these steps can help reduce the incidence of breast cancer-related mortality in Nigeria.

Prof. Erhabor Osaro (PhD.)
Manchester, United Kingdom

Acknowledgement

My sincere thanks goes to AuthorHouse Publishers UK, for their assistance and contribution to the publication of this book; to my Father in the Lord, Bishop David O. Oyedepo for being an inspiration in my life through his teachings; to Pastor Timi Davies for his spiritual oversight; not forgotten my Parents Late Mr Aibangbee and Mrs Rose Erhabor; to my co-labourers in the fight against breast cancer in Nigeria; Retsky Michael, Demicheli Romano, Forget Patrice, Vaidya Jayant, Bello Shaibu, Adias Teddy Charles, Dagana Amos, Egenti Nonye B, Mainasara Abdullah Suleiman, Sahabi SM, Rilwanu TI, Ahmed Yakubu, Hassan Mairo, Bashir Bello and Ifedayo Ajayi. I also wish to thank my wife; Mrs Angela Erhabor and my children; Emmanuel, Majesty, David, Daniel and Michelle. To the source of my life and strength, the Almighty God be all the praise.

Table of Contents

Chapter	Title	Page Number
	Preface	vii
	Acknowledgement	ix
1.	Introduction	1
2.	Challenge of Suboptimal Access to Mastectomy	12
3.	Lack of Access to Optimum Mammography and other Diagnostic Services	17
4.	Challenges associated with Access to radiotherapy and chemotherapy treatment	25
5.	Challenge Associated with Screening for Breast Cancer in Nigeria	30
6.	Late stage breast cancer among premenopausal Nigerian women	38
7.	Challenge of Triple Negative Brest Cancer (TNBC) in Nigeria	48
8.	Challenges Associated with Carrying out Randomized Clinical Trials on Breast Cancer in Nigeria	57
9.	Failure in Stewardship in the Management of Breast Cancer by the Nigerian Government	65
10.	Socioeconomic Factors and Unaffordability of Breast Cancer Treatment in Nigeria.	70

11.	Challenge of Increasing Incidence of Risk Factors for Breast Cancer in Nigeria	77
12.	Challenge of Poor Awareness of Breast Self Examination (BSE)	86
13.	Role of Spirituality in the Delay in Seeking Care among Breast Cancer Patients	92
14.	Challenge of Increasing Incidence of Breast Cancer among Men	97
15.	Poor knowledge and awareness- related challenges associated with Breast Cancer	105
16.	Lack of access to diagnostic test to determine predisposition to Breast Cancer	110
17.	Poor access to Breast Cancer diagnostic services in rural settings	117
18.	Pregnancy and breast cancer in Nigeria	124
INDEX		129

Chapter 1

Introduction

Breast Cancer constitutes a major public health issue globally, with over 1 million new cases diagnosed annually; resulting in over 400,000 annual deaths and about 4.4 million women living with the disease. It also affects one in eight women during their lives. It is the commonest site specific malignancy affecting women and the most common cause of cancer mortality in women worldwide. Breast cancer is a malignant (cancerous) growth that begins in the tissues of the breast. Cancer is a disease in which abnormal cells grow in an uncontrolled way. It is the most common cancer in women, but it can also appear in men. Breast cancer is now an epidemic, posing a serious threat to the health of women of all races globally. In Nigeria, cervical cancer was the commonest cause of cancer- related deaths among women for several decades but breast cancer is now the leading cause of cancer related deaths among Nigerian women. This is not due to a reduction in cervical cancer but an increase in the incidence of breast cancer. Breast cancer is commonly seen in four stages that represents its progression.

In stage I, the disease is confined entirely to the breast. The cancer usually start as a very tiny growth that cannot yet be felt but can be detected with imaging tests such as mammography and ultrasound. At this first stage, treatment is usually curative and more than 95% of those so detected will survive the disease beyond 5 years. Stage II is a cancer that has involved lymph nodes in the armpit of the same side of the breast, while stage III disease is one that has involved the muscles under the breast. Stages II and III therefore require very aggressive treatment using different modalities to contain the spread of the disease. It is however difficult to cure a patient in stage IV because the disease has spread and may have involved other organs in the body such as the lungs, liver, bones, the brain or the spine.

The five year survival rate for breast cancer patients in the United States exceeds 85%, in Nigeria it is a dismal 10%. Breast cancer is responsible for about 16% of all cancer related deaths in Nigeria [1].

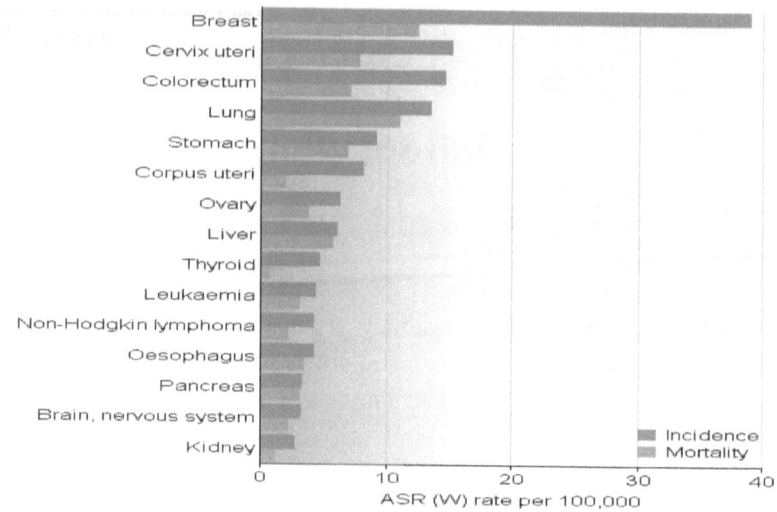

Figure 1: WHO statistics on Cancer among women

There are many risk factors that have been associated with breast cancer. Being a female, the risk increases with the age of the woman; the older a woman, the increased chances of getting breast cancer. History of breast cancer in close relatives especially in mothers and siblings has been associated with the risks of getting breast cancer, early onset of menstrual periods before the age of 12 years or reaching menopause after the age of 55 years has both been associated with risks of developing breast cancer, prolonged period of estrogen exposure in females, overweight, using hormone replacement therapy, taking birth control pills, drinking alcohol, not having children or having your first child after age 35 or having dense breasts.

The incidence of cancers is increasing worldwide. A steady increase in incidence has been observed in most developed and developing countries. Apart from incidence, cancer related deaths are also increasing. In 2008 alone, about 7.6 million people died from cancers globally, with about 70% of these deaths occurring in developing countries. In Nigeria, it is estimated that more than 250,000 new cases of cancers are diagnosed every year, and up to 10,000 Nigerians die each year from cancer related causes. These estimates may not be a reflection of the true picture as they are often largely based on hospital generated data without provision for the many cases that do not present in hospitals, those managed by traditional medicine practitioners, as well as the many cases of misdiagnosis in our numerous peripheral hospitals. There are over 230,000 new cases of breast cancer each year in the United States as of 2015. About 40,000 fatalities occur in the U.S. every year from this particular form of cancer[2]. The risk of breast cancer increases with age, and in the U.S. approximately one out of eight women will get breast cancer at some point in their lives. The physical, emotional and financial cost of this disease is staggering.

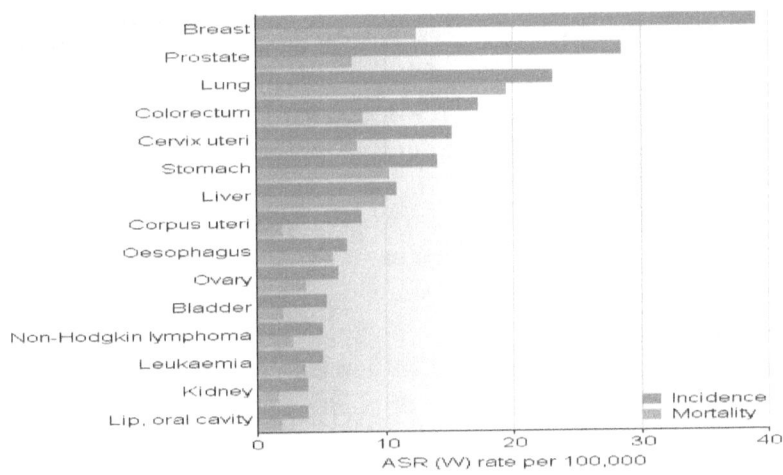

Figure 2: WHO statistics on Cancer among both gender (WHO, 2011)

The incidence of cancer continues to rise all over the world, and current projections show that there will be 1.27 million new cases and almost 1 million deaths by 2030. In view of the rising incidence of cancer in sub Saharan Africa (SSA), urgent steps are needed to guide appropriate policy, health sector investment and resource allocation. Information provided by Hospital Based Cancer Registry (HBCR) is beneficial and can be utilized for the improvement of cancer care delivery systems in low and middle income countries where there are no population based cancer registries.[3] Worldwide, more than one million new cases of female breast cancer are diagnosed each year, making it the most commonly occurring disease in women, accounting for over 1/3 of the estimated annual 4.7million cancer diagnosis in females and the second most common tumour after lung cancer in both sexes.[4] It is also the most common female cancer in both developed and developing countries with 55% of it occurring in the developing countries.[5] In addition, the annual worldwide incidences has almost doubled since 1975 and the prevalence and incidences increased with increasing age.[6] Death rates of 76/100,000 females is estimated to occur in 2020. Research has shown that life time risk of this disease nearly tripled within 50 years as 1 in 20 women had it in 1960, and 1 in every 7 in 1980. However since 1987, breast cancer rates increased by 0.5% each year and between 85% and 90% of the cases cannot be attributed to inherited genetic predisposition.[7] The age standardized incidence rates for breast cancer in the period 1960–1969 was 13.7 per 100 000 and it rose to 24.7 per 100 000 by 1998–1999; more or less a doubling of incidence over 4 decades or approximately 25% increase in incidence per decade.[8] With incidence in 2009 to 2010 at 54.3 per 100 000, this represents a 100% increase in the last decade. This is supported by the literature showing a rise in breast cancer incidence rates in sub Saharan Africa.[9-10]

Cancer has become a major source of morbidity and mortality globally.[11] In 2008, there were 12.7 million new cases and 7.6 million cancer related deaths.[12] A majority of the 56% of newly reported cancer cases occurred in developing countries and it is projected that by 2030, 70% of all new cases of cancer will be found in developing countries.[13] Most of this increase in incidence is a result of population growth and increased life expectancy.[14] Breast cancer is the number one cancer killer of Nigerian women. The steady rise in breast cancer cases in Nigeria is an indication of inadequate or ineffective control measures to curtail the disease or possibly due to diversion of global attention to HIV/AIDS and tuberculosis in the country. In Nigeria, some 100,000 new cases of cancer occur every year, with high case fatality ratio.[12] With approximately 20% of the population of Africa and slightly more than half the population of West Africa, Nigeria contributed 15% to the estimated 681,000 new cases of cancer that occurred in Africa in 2008.[11] Similar to the situation in the rest of the developing world, a significant proportion of the increase in incidence of cancer in Nigeria is due to increasing life expectancy, reduced risk of death from infectious diseases, increasing prevalence of smoking, physical inactivity, obesity, as well as changing dietary and lifestyle patterns. Despite the threat that cancer poses to public health in sub Saharan Africa, few countries in this region have data on cancer incidence. Most of the cancer incidence data in SSA in recent times is based on reports from registries in Gambia, Zimbabwe and Uganda.[15] These cancer registries have consistently provided incidence data for the last 10–20 years despite the difficulties of sustaining cancer registration in developing countries.[16-20] Breast cancer in the African continent is characterized by regional variation, as the incidence was 27% in North African countries (Algeria and Egypt) compared with 15% in sub Saharan Africa.[21] Breast cancer is a very common disease in Nigeria. It is often associated with a poor prognosis for a variety of reasons.[22-24] A study that investigated the level of occurrence and pattern of distribution of different cancer types in two major functional cancer registries in South-Western Nigeria showed a total number of 5,094 cancer patients registered between 2005 and 2009 in both Lagos (60%) and Ibadan (40%) cancer registries. Breast cancer accounted for the majority of cases (20.2%).[25] A retrospective review data of breast cancers between 2001 and 2005 in the University of Maiduguri Teaching Hospital Cancer Registry involving a total of 1,216 cases of cancers showed that breast cancer accounted for 13.9%.[26] In the North Western geopolitical zone of Nigeria, cancer of the breast was second to cancer of the cervix, while at University College Hospital (UCH), Ibadan (situated in the South Western geopolitical zone of Nigeria), it was the leading malignancy among women.[27] In the North Central geopolitical zone, breast cancer constituted 22.41% of new cancer cases registered in 5 years and accounted for 35.41% of all cancers in women.[10] In developing or low income countries, breast cancer is characterized by late clinical presentation and advance stages of the disease, when only chemotherapy and palliative care could be offered, and therefore associated with high mortality.[28,29]

The prevalence of non-communicable diseases including cancers is on the increase in developing countries.[30] With scientific development, better healthcare facilities and gradual decline in mortality, people are living longer and the population is gradually ageing. This has brought about an increasing incidence in non-communicable diseases including breast cancer worldwide. The prognosis is however worse in developing compared to developed countries.[31] An estimated 212,920 new cases of invasive breast cancer, 61,980 in situ cases, and 40,970 deaths were expected to occur among US women in 2006.[32] It is estimated that 1 in 8 Caucasian women (1 in 14 African American) in the US, and 1 in 12 in Britain will develop cancer of the breast in their life time.[33] Breast cancer is fast becoming one of the commonest cancer affecting women in Nigeria.[34-36] A previous report indicates that 1 in 5 (23%) case of breast mass diagnosed in Zaria is malignant in nature.[37] The overall survival rate among Nigerian women with breast cancer is low and patients with early breast cancer tend to have better survival than those with advanced disease. The majority of breast cancer patients in Nigeria tend to be young pre-menopausal women with advanced breast cancer.[38] Most Afro-Caribbean women are not as fortunate as their counterparts in the developed world. They are more likely to be diagnosed with advanced breast cancer.[39] The overall survival rate is 70.4% at 36 months among African women compared to a survival rate of 95% and above seen among women in developed economies.[32] Unlike developing countries, survival rates for breast cancer in developed countries have been improving in the last 20 years and more women are being successfully treated than ever before.[40] Management of patients with breast cancer is a major challenge to physicians in Nigeria and other developing countries. There are many factors that play a role in the poor prognosis of women with breast cancer in Nigeria; lack of advanced technology (diagnosis and monitoring), late presentation of patients to the hospital, poor access to cancer medication and the aggressive characteristics of breast cancers seen among Nigerian women, patronage of traditional healers who put incisions on the breast lesion perhaps causing more metastasis, ignorance due to lack of awareness and poor education and poverty.[41-46]

References

1. Okobia M.N, Bunker C.H, Okonofua FE, Osime U. Knowledge, attitude and practice of Nigerian women towards breast cancer: A cross-sectional study. *World Journal of Surgical Oncology* 2006; 4: 11–15.

2. *Cancer Facts & Figures.* Annual publication of the American Cancer Society, Atlanta, Georgia (2013):1-64.

3. Jedy-Agba EE, Curado MP, Oga E, Samaila MO, Ezeome ER, Obiorah C, Erinomo OO, Ekanem IO, Uka C, Mayun A, Afolayan EA, Abiodun P, Olasode BJ, Omonisi A, Otu T, Osinubi P, Dakum P, Blattner W, Adebamowo CA. The role of hospital-based cancer

registries in low and middle income countries-The Nigerian Case Study. Cancer Epidemiology. 2012;36(5):430-435.

4. Cancer Statistics Worldwide (2005). *London Cancer Research Report* (No.104).

5. Adetifa Felicia A., Ojikutu, Rasheed K. Prevalence and Trends in Breast Cancer in Lagos State, Nigeria. *African Research Review 2009; 3 (5): 1-15.*

6. Althuis, M.D., Dozier, J. M., Anderson, W.F., Devesa, S.S., Brinton, L.A. *Global Trends in Breast Cancer and Mortality; 1973-1997. Int. Journal of Epidemiology. 2005:---.*

7. American Cancer Society. Breast Cancer Facts & Figures 2013-2014; 37.

8. Parkin DM, Hamdi-Chérif M, Sitas F, Thomas JO, Wabinga H, Whelan SL, editors. Cancer In Africa IARC Scientific Publication No 153. 2003.

9. Forouzanfar MH, Foreman KJ, Delossantos AM, Lozano R, Lopez AD, Murray CJ, Naghavi M. Breast and cervical cancer in 187 countries between 1980 and 2010: a systematic analysis. Lancet. 2011.

10. Afolayan EAO, Ibrahim OOK, Ayilara GT. Cancer Patterns In Ilorin: An Analysis Of Ilorin Cancer Registry Statistics. *The Tropical Journal of Health Sciences.* 2012; 9:42-47.

11. Sylla BS, Wild CP. A million Africans a year dying from cancer by 2030: What can cancer research and control offer to the continent? Int J Cancer. 2011.

12. Ferlay J, Shin HR, Bray F, Forman D, Mathers C, Parkin DM. Estimates of worldwide burden of cancer in 2008: GLOBOCAN 2008. Int J Cancer. 2010; 127:2893–2917.

13. Boyle P, Levin B. International Agency for Research on Cancer. World Cancer Report 2008; Lyon, France. 2008.2008.

14. Lyerly HK, Abernethy AP, Stockler MR, Koczwara B, Aziz Z, Nair R, Seymour L. Need for Global Partnership in Cancer Care: Perceptions of Cancer Care Researchers Attending the 2010 Australia and Asia Pacific Clinical Oncology Research Development Workshop. J Oncol Pract. 2011; 7:324–329.

15. Curado MP, Edwards B, Storm H, Ferlay J, Heanue M, Boyle P, editors. Cancer Incidence in Five Continents. IARC Scientific Publications No 160. 2008 IX.

16. Chokunonga BME, Chirenje ZM, Nyabakau AM, Parkin DM. Cancer Survival in Zimbabwe 1993–1997. IARC Scientific Publication. 2011; 2011(162):249–255.

17. Chokunonga E, Levy LM, Bassett MT, Borok MZ, Mauchaza BG, Chirenje MZ, Parkin DM. Aids and cancer in Africa: the evolving epidemic in Zimbabwe. AIDS. 1999;13: 2583–2588.

18. Bah E, Sam O, Whittle H, Ramanakumar A, Sankaranarayanan R. Cancer survival in the Gambia, 1993–1997. IARC Sci Publ. 2011:97–100.

19. Parkin DM, Wabinga H, Nambooze S, Wabwire-Mangen F. AIDS-related cancers in Africa: maturation of the epidemic in Uganda. AIDS. 1999; 13:2563–2570.

20. Wabinga H, Parkin DM, Nambooze S, Amero J. Cancer survival in Kampala, Uganda, 1993–1997. IARC Sci Publ. 2011:243–247.

21. Parkin DM. Global cancer statistics in the year 2000. Lancet Oncol. 2001;2(9):533-543.

22. Adesunkanmi AR, Lawal OO, Adelusola KA, Durosimi MA. The severity, outcome and challenges of breast cancer in Nigeria. *Breast*. 2006; 15:399–409.

23. Irabor DO, Okolo CA. Outcome of one hundred and forty-nine consecutive breast biopsies in Ibadan, Nigeria. Breast Dis. 2011; 33(3):109-114.

24. Mayun AA, Obiano SK, Shehu SK, Abdulazeez JO. Breast malignancies in a tertiary health setting in north-eastern Nigeria: a histopathological review. Afr J Med Med Sci. 2009;38(4):337-341.

25. Awodele O, Adeyomoye AA, Awodele DF, Fayankinnu VB, Dolapo DC. Cancer distribution pattern in south-western Nigeria. Tanzan J Health Res. 2011 ; 13(2):125-131.

26. Nggada HA, Yawe KD, Abdulazeez J, Khalil MA. Breast cancer burden in Maiduguri, North eastern Nigeria. Breast J. 2008;14(3):284-286.

27. Afolayan EAO. Cancer in North Western region of Nigeria - an update analysis of Zaria cancer registry data. *Western Nig. Jour. of Med. Sci.* 2008; 1:37 – 43.

28. Adeniji KA. Pathological Appraisal of Carcinoma of the female breast in Ilorin, Nigeria. The Nigerian Postgraduate Medical Journal. 1999; 6: 56-59.

29. Anyanwu SNC Temporal Trends in Breast Cancer Presentation in the Third World UICC World Cancer Congress. Washington D C 2006.

30. Lucas AO, Gilles HM. Non-Communicable Disease: Health in Transition. In Short Textbook of Public Health Medicine for the Tropics. International Students Edition. Arnold Publishers 2003; 237-259.

31. Jemal A, Siegel R, Ward E, Murray T, Xu J, Smigal C, et al. Cancer statistics, 2006. CA Cancer J Clin. 2006;56(2):106-130.

32. Smigal C, Jemal A, Ward E, et al. Trends in breast cancer by race and ethnicity: update 2006. *CA Cancer Journal for Clinicians.* 2006; 56(3):168–183.

33. Badoe EA, Archampong EO, da Rocha-Afodu JT. The Breast. In Principles and Practice of Surgery including Pathology in the tropics. Third Ed. Ghana Publishing Corporation 2000; 457-477.

34. Afolayan EA. Five years of Cancer Registration at Zaria (1992 - 1996). Niger *Postgrad Med J.* 2004; 11(3):225-229.

35. Dogo D, Pindiga PU, Yawe T. Pattern of breast lesions in north eastern Nigeria. Tropical J Med Research 2000; 3:14-17.

36. Mandog BM. Obekpa, P.O. Orkar, K.S. Histopathological pattern of breast disease in Jos. Niger Postgrad Med J. 1998;5:167-170.

37. Yusufu LM, Odigie VI, Mohammed A. Breast Masses in Zaria. Ann Afr Med. 2003; 2: 13-16.

38. Terfa S. Kene, Vincent I. Odigie, Lazarus MD. Yusufu, Bidemi O. Yusuf, Sani M. Shehu, John T. Kase. Pattern of Presentation and Survival of Breast Cancer in a Teaching Hospital in North Western Nigeria. Oman Med J. 2010; 25(2): 104–107.

39. Ghafoor A, Jemal A, Ward E, et al. Trend in breast cancer by race and ethnicity. Cancer J Clin 2003; 53:342-355.

40. Jemal A, Tiwari RC, Murray T, et al. Cancer Statistics. Cancer J Clin 2004; 54:8-29.

41. Chlebowski RT, Chen Z, Anderson GL, et al. Ethnicity and breast cancer: Factors influencing differences in incidence and outcome. J Natl Cancer Inst. 2005; 97:439-448.

42. Odigie VI, Yusufu LM, Rafindadi A, da Rocha-Afodu JT. Breast cancer in Zaria. Nig J Surg 2003; 9:46-50.

43. Anyanwu SN. Breast cancer in eastern Nigeria: a ten year review. West Afr J Med 2000; 19(2):120-125.

44. Dezheng Huo, Francis Ikpatt, Andrey Khramtsov, Jean-Marie Dangou, Rita Nanda, James Dignam, Bifeng Zhang, Tatyana Grushko, Chunling Zhang, Olayiwola Oluwasola, David Malaka, Sani Malami, Abayomi Odetunde, Adewumi O. Adeoye, Festus Iyare, Adeyinka Falusi, Charles M. Perou, and Olufunmilayo I. Olopade. Population Differences in Breast Cancer: Survey in Indigenous African Women Reveals Over-Representation of Triple-Negative Breast Cancer. J Clin Oncol. 2009 Sep 20; 27(27): 4515–4521.

45. Hassan I, Mabogunje O. Cancer of the male breast in Zaria, Nigeria. *East African Medical Journal.* 1995; 72(7):457–458.

46. Chiedozi LC. Morbidity, mortality and survival in the management of cT (4 breast cancer in Nigeria. Ann Saudi Med. 1995; 15(3):227-230.

Chapter 2

Challenge of Suboptimal Access to Mastectomy

Mastectomy is a medical term for the surgical removal of cancerous tissues from one or both breast (partially or completely). Mastectomy is usually carried out to treat breast cancer. In some cases, women at high risk of breast cancer can have the operation as a prophylactic or preventive measure. In some cases, patients can choose to have lumpectomy which involves wide local excision of a small volume of breast tissue containing the tumor. Mastectomy and lumpectomy are local therapies for breast cancer because they target the area of the tumor, compared to systemic therapies (chemotherapy, immunotherapy and hormonal therapy).

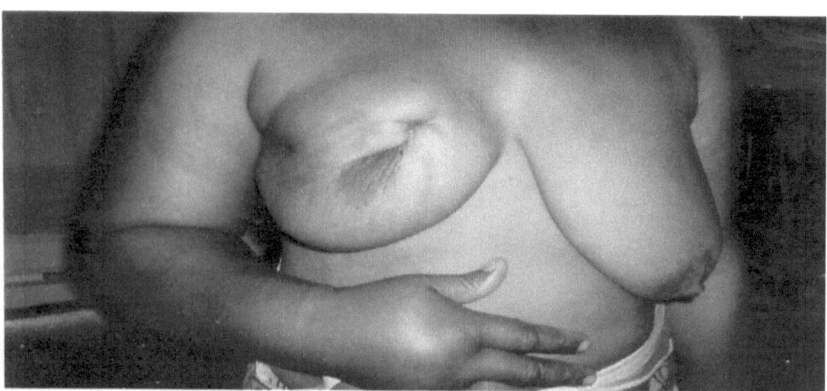

Figure 3: Lumpectomy in the right breast in a 50 years old Nigerian woman

The decision to carry out a mastectomy depends on a number of factors; breast size, number of lesions, biologic aggressiveness of the breast cancer and the availability of adjuvant radiation. Previous studies comparing mastectomy to lumpectomy with radiation have suggested that routine radical mastectomy surgeries cannot prevent later distant secondary tumors arising from micrometastases that had taken place prior to diagnosis and following surgery. Possible side effect associated with mastectomy include post-surgical pain, change in the shape of the breast(s), wound infection, haematoma (buildup of blood in the wound), and seroma (buildup of clear fluid in the wound). The surgical treatment of breast cancer has gone through phases. The early conservative excision gave way to Halsted's radical mastectomy and this, with its many modifications, became the traditional surgical treatment for over a century.[1-3] Modified radical mastectomy remains an important and essential component of the management of breast cancer, the increasing availability and utilization of adjuvant therapies notwithstanding. In a previous report on 2154 Nigerian breast cancer patients of all ages and socio-economic groups, 87% presented in stages III or IV and only 13% in stages I or II who were questioned on their reasons for not attending hospital sooner. The most common reason for delay (963 patients, 44.7%) was fear of mastectomy. Other reasons given include; preference for prayer houses or spiritual healing homes in 291 patients (13.5%), a belief that the lesion was inflammatory in 183 (8.5%), preference for native doctors or herbalists in 497 (23.1%) and economic reasons in 220 (10.2%).[4] Breast cancer in Nigeria is characterized by late presentation, younger age at diagnosis, large tumours and multiple nodal involvements. The pattern of presentation differs from that in the western world where most patients are post-menopausal and present with small sized early tumours and less aggressive disease.

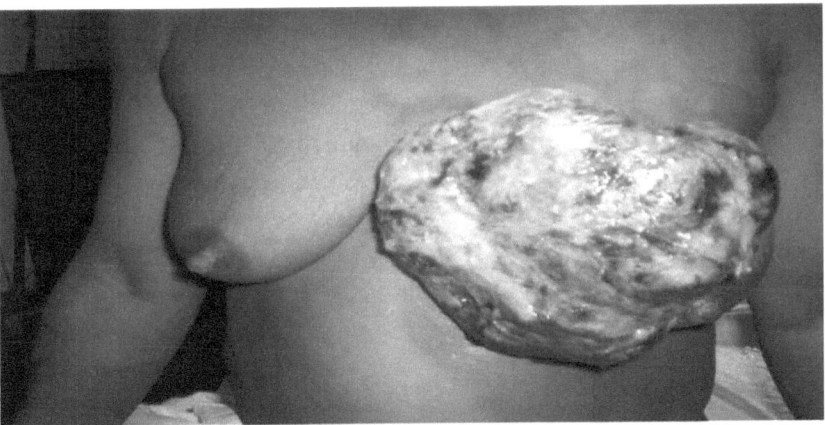

Figure 4: Mastectomy in a 48 years old Nigerian patient with Breast cancer

The use of conservative surgery as part of multidisciplinary management of breast cancer is increasing throughout the world. However complete surgical removal of the breast with its local lymphatic drainage remains the preferred surgical treatment in Nigeria and most low income countries (LICs) where breast conserving surgery is infrequently practiced. The reason for this disparity include; late stage of presentation, large size of tumours at diagnosis, lack of access to treatment, poor affordability and the aggressive nature of the disease commonly seen among Nigerian women and in other low income countries in sub Saharan Africa.[5-8] Breast conserving surgery in Nigeria and other settings in sub Saharan Africa is associated with many challenges including; logistics limitations such as poor access to radiotherapy services and inefficient follow-up programmes. Breast cancer surgery (BCS) rate is low in Nigeria and most developing countries compared to findings from more developed economies. Surveillance, Epidemiology, and End Results (SEER) data set which included 1,011 Metaplastic breast cancer (MBC) and 253,818 Infiltrating Ductal Carcinoma (IDC) patients in the US diagnosed from 2001 to 2010 indicated that MBC patients had larger, higher grade tumours, had less frequent axillary nodal involvement, and were more likely to be treated with mastectomy.[9] Records of 6,263 patients with resectable breast cancer admitted in a hospital in China from June 1963 to June 2003, were analyzed retrospectively. Breast cancer occurred most frequently in patients of 40-49 years old (41.0%) and especially in patients of 45-49 years old (25.2%). Breast lump was the main clinical manifestation, and occurred in 96.2% of the patients.[10] Similarly, among 9,670 patients operated on for primary breast cancer during the 16.5 years period from 1986 to 2002 at CIH Tokyo, Japan there were 2,449 patients who underwent breast conserving surgery (BCS).[11] This breast cancer surgery (BCS) rate in New Zealand in a previous study was 58.6% of patients over a 5 year period.[12] A total of 28,536 cases of female breast cancers were reported to the Missouri Cancer Registry and Research Centre between 2003 and 2008. Of these, 25 743 (90.2%) were Caucasian (White) while 2,793 (9.8%) were African-American (Black). Analysis showed that the proportion of African-Americans with late stage detection exceeded that of whites in almost all rural and urban locations.[13] Experience in a busy university college hospital in Nigeria involving 1,226 newly diagnosed breast cancer patients indicated that over the study period, 431 (35.2%) patients underwent mastectomy making an average of 43 mastectomies per year. Most patients were young women, premenopausal, had invasive ductal carcinoma and underwent modified radical mastectomy as the definitive surgical treatment.[14] The reasons for low mastectomy rate in Nigeria and other developing counties include; late presentation with inoperable local or metastatic tumours necessitating only palliative or terminal care, inability of a significant number of patients to pay out-of-pocket for treatment, unwillingness to have mastectomy because of the associated stigma associated with the disease, fear of being abandoned by their partners or of losing their jobs, illiteracy and erroneous religious beliefs often prevent women from having access to services.[14]

References

1. Hanagiri T, Nagata Y, Monji S, Shinohara S, Takenaka M, Shigematsu Y, Shimokawa H, Nakagawa M, Uramoto H, So T, Tanaka F. Temporal trends in the surgical outcomes of patients with breast cancer. World J Surg Oncol. 2012; 10:108.

2. Loukas M, Tubbs RS, Mirzayan N, Shirak M, Steinberg A, Shoja MM. The history of mastectomy. Am Surg. 2011; 77(5):566-571.

3. Singletary SE. Breast cancer management: the road to today. Cancer. 2008; 113(7):1844-1849.

4. Ajekigbe AT. Fear of mastectomy: The most common factor responsible for late presentation of carcinoma of the breast in Nigeria. *Clinical Oncology*; 1991; 3(2): 78–80.

5. Yip CH, Buccimazza I, Hartman M, Deo SV, Cheung PS. Improving outcomes in breast cancer for low and middle income countries. World J Surg. 2015; 39(3):686-92.

6. Ntirenganya F, Petroze RT, Kamara TB, Groen RS, Kushner AL, Kyamanywa P, Calland JF, Kingham TP. Prevalence of breast masses and barriers to care: results from a population-based survey in Rwanda and Sierra Leone. J Surg Oncol. 2014; 110(8):903-906.

7. Mody GN, Nduaguba A, Ntirenganya F, Riviello R. Characteristics and presentation of patients with breast cancer in Rwanda.Am J Surg. 2013; 205(4):409-413.

8. Malik AM, Pathan R, Shaikh NA, Qureshi JN, Talpur KA.Pattern of presentation and management of ca breast in developing countries. There is a lot to do. J Pak Med Assoc. 2010; 60(9):718-721.

9. Nelson RA, Guye ML, Luu T, Lai LL. Survival outcomes of metaplastic breast cancer patients: results from a US population-based analysis. Ann Surg Oncol. 2015; 22(1):24-31.

10. Yang MT, Rong TH, Huang ZF, Zeng CG, Long H, Fu JH, Lin P, Wang X, Wang SY, Wang X, Tang J.Clinical analysis of resectable breast cancer: a report of 6 263 cases. Ai Zheng. 2005; 24(3):327-331.

11. Kasumi F, Takahashi K, Nishimura S, Iijima K, Miyagi U, Tada K, Makita M, Iwase T, Oguchi M, Yamashita T, Akiyama F, Sakamoto G.CIH-Tokyo experience with breast-conserving surgery without radiotherapy: 6.5 year follow-up results of 1462 patients. Breast J. 2006; 12(5 Suppl 2):S181-190.

12. Lee DW, Vallance S. Surgical management of breast cancer in a small peripheral New Zealand hospital. ANZ J Surg. 2006; 13:1060–1063.

13. Williams F, Jeanetta S, O'Brien DJ, Fresen JL. Rural-urban difference in female breast cancer diagnosis in Missouri. Rural Remote Health. 2015; 15(3):3063.

14. Ogundiran TO, Ayandipo OO, Ademola AF, Adebamowo CA. Mastectomy for management of breast cancer in Ibadan, Nigeria. BMC Surg. 2013; 13:59.

Chapter 3

Lack of Access to Optimum Mammography and other Diagnostic Services

Mammography is the process of using low-energy X-rays (usually around 30 kVp) to examine the human breast. It can be used as a diagnostic and screening tool for breast cancer. The main aim of carrying out mammography is to allow for the early detection of breast cancer, allowing for timely intervention and prevention of secondary metastasis. For the average woman, the United States Preventive Services Task Force recommends that women between the ages of 50 and 74 have a mammography every two years.[1] The American College of Radiology and American Cancer Society recommend yearly screening mammography starting at the age of 40 years. Women in the UK aged between 50 and 70 are routinely invited every three years to have a test to look for early breast cancer.[2,3] The Canadian Task Force on Preventive Health Care and the European Cancer Observatory recommends mammography every 2–3 years between 50 and 69. Unlike most women in the West, a significant number of women in Nigeria and other developing countries are not as privileged. Accessibility and cost are major limiting factors why many African women cannot access this lifesaving screening. This may be one of the reasons, while many present to hospital at a late and more challenging stage with attendant poor prognosis. There is however advocacy that mammograms should not be done with increased frequency in people undergoing breast surgery, including breast enlargement, mastopexy, and breast reduction surgery.[4] Apart from unnecessary surgery and anxiety, there are risks associated with more frequent mammograms including a small but significant increase in breast cancer induced by radiation.[5] Previous report advocates that the time has come to reassess whether universal mammography screening should be recommended for any age group.[6] Some school of thought advocates that it may no longer be reasonable to attend breast cancer screening at any age but rather at an age when it is clinically indicated. Mammography has a false negative (missed cancer) rate of at least 10 percent. This is partly due to dense tissues obscuring the cancer and the fact that the appearance of cancer on mammograms has a large overlap with the appearance of normal tissues.[7-9]

The use of mammography as a screening tool for the detection of early breast cancer in otherwise healthy women without symptoms is controversial.[7-8] Previous report indicates that a significant number of women will suffer from significant psychological stress due to false positive results, overtreatment and radiation exposure.[10] Similarly it has been reported that mammography does not reduce death overall, but causes significant harm by inflicting cancer scare and unnecessary surgical interventions.[11] Repeated mammography starting at age 50 has been shown to save about 1.8 lives over 15 years for every 1,000 women screened.[12] It is not really clear whether screening does more good than harm. There seems a consensus in most developed countries that the potential risks of routine screening for healthy women might outweigh the benefits.[7] Of every 1,000 women who are screened in the United States of America, about 10%–15% will be called back for a diagnostic session. About 10 of these individuals will be referred for a biopsy; the remaining 60 are found to be of benign cause. Of the 10 referred for biopsy, about 3.5 will have a cancer and 6.5 will not. Of the 3.5 who have cancer, about 2 have a low stage cancer that will be essentially cured after treatment. The disadvantages of using mammogram as a screening tool for the detection of early breast cancer in otherwise healthy women include; over-diagnosis (detection of breast cancers through screening that would not have been diagnosed without screening and would not have threatened the lives of the women concerned), false positive mammograms can lead to unnecessary further investigations, can produce a false reassurance due to missed cancer and incorrect diagnosis, cause pain and discomfort associated with mammography, psychological distress and the risk of exposure to radiation which in itself can potentially increase the risk of breast cancer.[13-17]

Mammograms also have a rate of missed tumors (false negatives). Estimates of the false negative rate depend on close follow-up of a large number of patients for many years. This is difficult in practice particularly in Nigeria and other developing countries because many women do not return for regular mammography, making it impossible to know if they ever developed a cancer. Women aged 40 to 49 have one in four instances of cancer missed at each mammography.[18] The reason for false negative mammogram is that breast tissue particularly among younger women is denser thus making it difficult to detect tumors. A group of 3,184 women had mammograms which were formally classified as probably benign. Follow up 6 monthly biopsy for the next 3 indicated that of these 3,184 women, 17 (0.5%) did have cancers. However, when these diagnosis was made, they were all still in the early stage (0 or 1). Five years after treatment, none of these 17 women had evidence of recurrence. This is an indication that small early cancers, even though not acted on immediately may still be entirely curable.[19]

There are four categories of cancers found by mammography; cancers that are so easily treated that a later detection would have produced the same total cure (woman would have lived even without mammography); cancers so aggressive that even early detection is too late (woman dies despite detection by mammography); cancers that would have receded on their own or are so slow-growing that the woman would die of other causes before the cancer produces symptoms (mammography results in over diagnosis and over treatment of this class) and the small number of breast cancers that are detected by screening mammography and whose treatment outcome improves as a result of earlier detection. Only between 3% and 13% of breast cancers detected by screening mammography will fall into this last category. The goal of any screening procedure is to examine a large population of patients and find the small number most likely to have a serious condition. False positive mammograms however may affect a woman's well-being and behavior. Some women who receive false positive results may be more likely to return for routine screening or perform breast self examinations more frequently. However, some women who receive false positive results become anxious, worried and distressed about the possibility of having breast cancer, feelings that can last for many years. False positives mammogram has a number of implications; it means greater expense, both for the individual woman and for the screening program. With follow-up screening typically much more expensive than initial screening, more false positives tend to receive more follow-up testing that can potentially result in fewer women having access, particularly in the Nigerian setting where access and funding is naturally limited.

Lack of access to diagnostic and radiography equipment and radiotherapy equipment, particularly for rural women. There are few functioning mammogram equipment to cater for the highly populated Nigerian nation (almost 160 million people). Most developed countries with less population of about 8 million have more than 8 dozen centres for radiation therapy, and about a hundred specialists in radiation therapy. However, in Nigeria with a population of greater than 160 million people, less than 10 centres have facilities for radiation therapy and most of the times only 3 or 4 are functional leading to overcrowding and patients having to travel hundreds of kilometres for radiation therapy. Evidenced- based best practice in the developed world has shown that hospitals may not always be the best places to treat cancer patients in developing countries, particularly when long-term chemotherapy schedules may require women to travel far from home and their families (community treatment centres may be the way forward in developing countries).

On the other hand, Mammography, a form of X-ray of the breast, is able to detect growth or changes in the breast that are still very tiny as not to be felt by hand examination of even the expert. If abnormal findings are seen on the films, attention can then be directed to the area for further tests. Any cancer detected and treated at such an early stage when it is not yet large enough to be felt has a very high chance of total cure. The common belief among Nigerians is that breast cancer is only a disease of women and it cannot affect men. The disease however affects men, and 1-2% of breast cancers may occur in the rudimentary breasts in men. In most instances, the affected men do not seek treatment for the swelling early due to poor knowledge. Evidence from previous report indicates that among men with breast cancer, it is often difficult to convince the relations of male breast cancer patient about the need for treatment since they commonly believe it is a "boil" that is persisting. Breast imaging plays a vital role in the multidisciplinary approach to management of breast disease. The level of awareness of breast cancer is quite high, with the positive mammographic yield emphasizing the value of a multidisciplinary approach in the management of breast diseases.[20-21] There is low level of awareness about mammography and mammographic screening in Nigeria, indicating the need to educate women about the risk of breast cancer and the importance of screening as a tool for the early detection and treatment of this condition.[22] There are various documentations on findings in breast cancer screening programmes mostly from countries[23-25] with established screening programmes with relatively scanty reports from developing countries.[26-28] Increased awareness of breast cancer and recent establishment of some breast imaging units in Nigeria has led to high turnout of patients.

Tempering the strong suggestions that mammography should be more used in developing countries, there are other reasons to suggest the contrary – that mammography has not been successful in reducing the breast cancer problem in developed countries and has in fact made it worse. This is particularly true for women aged 40-49 [29]. However there may be an optimal solution to this issue. Retsky and colleagues [29] attributes the lack of benefit and harm in some cases of early detection of breast cancer in women 40-49 to surgery driven angiogenesis of dormant micro metastases. However in a later paper [30], the same authors report that perioperative NSAID should curtail the surgery driven metastatic activity. Putting these findings together, what seems to make sense is to use both early detection and perioperative NSAID but not just early detection. That could be tested in a clinical trial among women of African descent. In addition, another consideration when discussing early diagnosis is that the use of survival data rather than mortality data (including all-cause mortality) may distort results in favor of early detection due to over-diagnosis and lead time bias.

References

1. *United States Preventive Services Task Force.* Breast Cancer Screening 2009.

2. NICE (2006) Familial breast cancer: the classification and care of women at risk of familial breast cancer in primary, secondary and tertiary care (partial update of NICE clinical guideline 14). *Replaced by CG164.* Clinical guideline 41.

3. Advisory Committee on Breast Cancer Screening (2006) Screening for breast cancer in England: past and future. NHS Cancer Screening Programmes.

4. American Society of Plastic Surgeons. Five Things Physicians and Patients Should Question", Choosing Wisely: an initiative of the ABIM Foundation (American Society of Plastic Surgeons), retrieved 25 July 2014.

5. Friedenson B. "Is mammography indicated for women with defective BRCA genes? Implications of recent scientific advances for the diagnosis, treatment, and prevention of hereditary breast cancer. *Med Gen Med. 2000;* 2 (1): E9. PMID 11104455.

6. Gøtzsche PC, Jørgensen KJ. Screening for breast cancer with mammography". *Cochrane Database Syst Rev. 2013;* 6 (6): CD001877.

7. Biller-Andorno, Nikola. Abolishing Mammography Screening Programs? A View from the Swiss Medical Board". *The New England Journal of Medicine.* 2014; 370: 1965–1967.

8. Pace LE, Keating NL. "A systematic assessment of benefits and risks to guide breast cancer screening decisions". JAMA 2014; 311 (13): 1327–1335.

9. Blausen Gallery. *Wikiversity Journal of Medicine.2014. Blausen.com staff.* DOI:10.15347/wjm/2014.010

10. Gøtzsche PC, Nielsen M. "Screening for breast cancer with mammography". *Cochrane Database Syst Rev. 2011;* (1): CD001877.

11. David H. Newman. *Hippocrates' Shadow.* Scibner 2008: 193. ISBN 1-4165-5153-0.

12. Nick Mulcahy. Screening Mammography Benefits and Harms in Spotlight Again". *Medscape.* April 2, 2009.

13. Duffy, S.W., Tabar, L., Olsen, A.H. et al. Absolute numbers of lives saved and overdiagnosis in breast cancer screening, from a randomized trial and from the Breast Screening Programme in England. *Journal of Medical Screening 2010;* 17(1), 25-30.

14. Gram, I.T., Lund, E. and Slenker, S.E. Quality of life following a false positive mammogram. *British Journal of Cancer 1990;* 62(6): 1018-1022.

15. Lerman, C., Trock, B., Rimer, B.K. et al. Psychological and behavioral implications of abnormal mammograms. *Annals of Internal Medicine* 1991; 114(8), 657-661.

16. Rutter, D.R., Calnan, M., Vaile, M.S. et al. Discomfort and pain during mammography: description, prediction, and prevention. *British Medical Journal. 1992;* 305(6851): 443-445.

17. Moss, S.M., Cuckle, H., Evans, A. et al. Effect of mammographic screening from age 40 years on breast cancer mortality at 10 years' follow-up: a randomised controlled trial. *Lancet 2006;* 368(9552): 2053-2060.

18. Epstein, S. S. (1978). *The Politics of Cancer*, San Francisco: Sierra Club Books. Abridged Japanese translation, 1978. Revised and expanded edition, Anchor/Doubleday Press, New York, 1979. *The Politics of Cancer, Revisited*, East Ridge Press, Fremont Center, N.Y., 1998.

19. Sickles A. Periodic. Mammographic Follow-up. Radiology 1991; 179:463-468.

20. Akande HJ, Olafimihan BB, Oyinloye OI. A five year audit of mammography in a tertiary hospital, North Central Nigeria. *Niger Med J.* 2015;56(3):213-217.

21. Obajimi MO, Ajayi IO, Oluwasola AO, Adedokun BO, Adeniji-Sofoluwe AT, Mosuro OA, Akingbola TS, Bassey OS, Umeh E, Soyemi TO, Adegoke F, Ogungbade I, Ukaigwe C, Olopade OI. Level of awareness of mammography among women attending outpatient clinics in a teaching hospital in Ibadan, South-West Nigeria. BMC Public Health. 2013; 16:13:40.

22. Akinola R, Wright K, Osunfidiya O, Orogbemi O, Akinola O. Mammography and mammographic screening: are female patients at

a teaching hospital in Lagos, Nigeria, aware of these procedures? *Diagn Interv Radiol.* 2011; 17(2):125-129.

23. Frisell J, Eklund G, Hellstrom L, Lidbrink E, Rutqvist LE, Somell A. Randomized study of mammography screening - preliminary report on mortality in the Stockholm trial. Breast Cancer Res Treat. 1991; 18:49–56.

24. Poplack SP, Tosteson AN, Grove MR, Wells WA, Carney PA. Mammography in 53,803 women from the New Hampshire mammography network. Radiology. 2000; 217:832–40.

25. Roberts MM, Alexander FE, Anderson TJ, Chetty U, Donnan PT, Forrest P, et al. Edinburgh trail of screening for breast cancer: Mortality at seven years. Lancet. 1990; 335:241–246.

26. Adesunkanmi AR, Agbakwuru EA. Benign breast disease at Wesley Guild Hospital, Ilesha, Nigeria. West Afr J Med. 2001; 20:146–51.

27. Irabor AO, Okolo CA. An audit of 149 consecutive breast biopsies in Ibadan, Nigeria. Pak J Med Sci. 2008; 24:257–262.

28. Ochicha O, Edino ST, Mohammed AZ, Amin SN. Benign breast lesions in Kano. Nig J Surg Res. 2002;4:1–5.

29. Retsky MW, Demicheli R, Hrushesky WJ, Baum M, Gukas ID. Dormancy and surgery-driven escape from dormancy help explain some clinical features of breast cancer. APMIS. 2008 Jul-Aug;116(7-8):730-41.

30. Retsky MW, Demicheli R, Hrushesky WJM, Forget P, DeKock M, Gukas I, Rogers RA, Baum M, Sukhatme V, Vaidya JS. Reduction of breast cancer relapses with perioperative non-steroidal anti-inflammatory drugs: new findings and a review. Current Medicinal Chemistry. 2013;20(33):4163-4176.

Chapter 4

Challenges associated with access to radiotherapy, chemotherapy and treatment

Radiotherapy (also known as radiation therapy) involves the use of high energy radiation, usually x-rays, to damage cancer cells and treat tumours in the breast. It has two equally important goals: to control the growth of the tumour and to do so while minimizing exposure to the surrounding normal, healthy tissue. Radiation therapy has an important role in treating all stages of breast cancer (stage 0 through stage III) after lumpectomy or mastectomy, because it is so effective and relatively safe. Radiation can also be very helpful to people with stage IV cancer that has spread to other parts of the body. Radiation therapy may be recommended after mastectomy to destroy any breast calls that may remain at the mastectomy site. Factors associated with a high risk of recurrence after mastectomy for which radiation may be indicated include; larger lump ($\geq$ 5 centimeters), a series of lumps, cancer that has invaded the lymph channels and blood vessels in the breast., one or more lymph nodes involvement, and in cases where the cancer has invaded the skin. Patients with these risk factors have a 20% to 30% risk of recurrence after mastectomy without radiation therapy. Radiation therapy would be recommended to help reduce this risk by up to 70% (for example, a 30% risk may be reduced to just under 10%). Treatment is given to the area where the breast used to be and sometimes to the lymph node regions nearby. Radiation is often contraindicated in; a patients who has had radiation to that area of the body before, where there is connective tissue disease (scleroderma or vasculitis), pregnancy, and patients who are not committed to the daily schedule of radiation therapy. Radiation may be given immediately after surgery or after other forms of treatment. Some examples of treatment sequences involving radiation; surgery followed by radiation and then possibly hormonal therapy, surgery followed by chemotherapy, then radiation and possibly hormonal therapy, and chemotherapy followed by targeted or hormonal therapy then surgery, radiation and possibly hormonal therapy. Newer technologies used in the West such as Intensity Modulated Radiotherapy (IMRT), Image Guided Radiotherapy (IGRT), Volumetric Arc Therapy (VMAT) and Stereotactic Body Radiotherapy (SBRT) are often beyond the reach of many patients in Nigeria and other developing countries. Intraoperative radiation (TARGIT) is potentially an improvement and is under active investigation in some countries.[1]

Chemotherapy is treatment with cancer-killing drugs that are given intravenously or orally. The drugs travel through the bloodstream to reach cancer cells in remote parts of the body. Chemotherapy is given in cycles, with each period of treatment followed by a recovery period. Chemotherapy can be given after surgery as adjuvant therapy to get rid of any residual cancer cells. The use of adjuvant chemotherapeutics after mastectomy reduces the risk of residual disease. Radiotherapy, chemotherapy, targeted therapy, and hormone therapy can all be used as adjuvant treatments in breast cancer. Chemotherapy can be given before surgery (neoadjuvant chemotherapy), can be given for large breast cancer lesions and advanced breast cancers. The aim of neoadjuvant chemotherapy is to possibly shrink the tumour so that it can be removed by less extensive and invasive surgery. Adjuvant and neoadjuvant treatments are most effective when combinations of more than one drug are used. Achieving local and distant disease control in locally advanced breast cancer (LABC), which may improve survival, remains a challenge. Neoadjuvant chemotherapy (NAC) has been demonstrated to be a helpful strategy in LABC, because of its tumour down staging benefits. [2-5] A previous report in Eastern Nigeria [5] revealed a low rate of adherence to NAC by patients. The reason for non-adherence included; lack of funds to procure chemotherapy and refusal of additional modality of treatment. [6] There are challenges associated with accessing breast radiation and chemotherapy treatment in Nigeria; most breast cancer patients often present with advanced breast cancer with high disease load on the breast and metastasis, available facilities are few and unevenly distributed, presence of old radiotherapy systems (Cobalt-60, EKOH, Linear accelerator); poor access and scheduling- related issues to radiation treatment in the few centres where facility is available, unaffordability of commonly used breast cancer chemotherapeutic agents like Doxorubicin, Epirubicin, CMF (Cyclophosphamide, Methotrexate and Fluorouracil), FAC (5-fluorouracil, Adriamycin (doxorubicin) and cyclophosphamide), Fluorouracil (5FU), AC (Adriamycin or doxorubicin and cyclophosphamide), AT (Adriamycin or doxorubicin and Paclitaxel (Taxol) or docetaxel (Taxotere). The most commonly used chemotherapy drugs in the developed world for early breast cancer include the; Anthracyclines (doxorubicin/Adriamycin), epirubicin/Ellence, Taxanes (paclitaxel/Taxol and docetaxel/Taxotere), Fluorouracil (5-FU), Cyclophosphamide (Cytoxan), Carboplatin, Trastuzumab (Herceptin) for cancers that are HER2 positive, Pertuzumab (Perjeta) can also be combined with trastuzumab and docetaxel for HER2 positive cancers. Commonly used chemotherapeutic drugs used in treating women with advanced breast cancer include; Docetaxel, Capecitabine (Xeloda), Paclitaxel, Liposomal doxorubicin (Doxil) Mitoxantrone Ixabepilone (Ixempra), Platinum agents (cisplatin, carboplatin), Vinorelbine (Navelbine), Gemcitabine (Gemzar), Albumin-bound paclitaxel (nab-paclitaxel or Abraxane) and Eribulin (Halaven). These potentially lifesaving chemotherapeutic agents are available to most breast cancer patients in the developed world. However they are often beyond the reach of a vast majority of women with breast cancer in Nigeria and other developing countries. This is a humanitarian issue of public health significance that will need to be addressed. Chemotherapy is associated with several effects. There is need to build the capacity of healthcare workers managing breast cancer patients in developing countries to effectively manage these side effects and optimize adherence. Some of the most common possible side effects include; hair loss and nail changes, mouth sores, loss of appetite or increased appetite, nausea and vomiting, pancytopenia (anaemia, leucopenia, neutropenia and thrombocytopenia), predisposition to infections, easy bruising or bleeding (thrombocytopenia), fatigue (anaemia), menstrual changes, infertility, neuropathy (taxanes, platinum agents, vinorelbine, erubulin, and ixabepilone), cardiomyopathy (doxorubicin and epirubicin), hand-foot syndrome (capecitabine and liposomal doxorubicin), chemo brain (observable decrease in mental functioning), increased risk of leukaemia (myelodysplastic syndrome and acute myeloid leukaemia), feeling unwell or tired and fatigue. Counselling facilities for patient to help with depression and encouragement for exercise, naps, and energy conserving strategies, sleep problems are often inadequate and sometimes not available. There is need to improve the access to chemotherapy and radiation treatment in Nigeria and other developing countries. Many low-resource countries have only 1 treatment machine for up to 10 million people. Some of the world's poorest nations have no radiotherapy facilities whatsoever. [7] Bringing the treatment closer to the patient, such as offering chemotherapy in local clinics, could be a better option. There are only a handful of radiation oncologists in Nigeria and other developing countries. As expected, this presents opportunities for corruption in accessing the service in the few tertiary hospitals with qualified radiation oncologists.

References

1. Vaidya JS, Bulsara M, Wenz F, Joseph D, Saunders C, Massarut S, Flyger H, Eiermann W, Alvarado M, Esserman L, Falzon M, Brew-Graves C, Potyka I, Tobias JS, Baum M; TARGIT trialists' group. Pride, Prejudice, or Science: Attitudes Towards the Results of the TARGIT-A Trial of Targeted Intraoperative Radiation Therapy for Breast Cancer. Int J Radiat Oncol Biol Phys. 2015 Jul 1;92(3):491-497.

2. Rastogi P, Anderson SJ, Bear HD, Geyer CE, Kahlenberg MS, Robidoux A, *et al.* Preoperative chemotherapy: Updates of National Surgical Adjuvant Breast and Bowel Project Protocol B-18 and B-27. J Clin Oncol 2008; 26:778-785.

3. Marafz R, Beross G, Svebis M, Gyanti R, Vizhanyo R, Hajnal L, *et al.* Response rates following neoadjuvant chemotherapy and breast preserving treatment in patients with locally advanced breast cancer. Magy Seb 2005; 58:225-32.

4. Beriwal S, Schwartz GF, Kumarnicky L, Garcia-Young JA. Breast conserving therapy after neoadjuvant chemotherapy: Long term results. Breast J 2006; 12:159-164.

5. Anyanwu SN, Egwuonwu OA, Ihekwoaba EC. Acceptance and adherence to treatment among breast cancer patients in Eastern Nigeria. Breast. 2011; 20 (2):S51-53.

6. Egwuonwu O A, Anyanwu S, Nwofor A. Default from neoadjuvant chemotherapy in premenopausal female breast cancer patients: What is to blame? Niger J Clin Pract 2012; 15:265-269.

Chapter 5

Challenge Associated with Screening for Breast Cancer in Nigeria

Screening programs are often used to test individuals who are asymptomatic, with the hope of identifying persons who are likely to have the disease of interest. Screening test may not be able to conclusively exclude the disease and may often require a supplemental test to further investigate those suspected, in a bid to confirm or exclude the disease. The main aim of breast cancer screening is to reduce risk of preventable deaths and improve the quality of life of the patients. Breast cancer detected early can be effectively treated, and at a cost effective cost.[1] From a public health point of view, screening test should only be implemented when the potential benefit of the screening outweigh the potential harm associated with the screening. Prevention and early detection are the major challenges associated with breast cancer management in Nigeria and other developing countries, despite being key to reduction of the incidence and severity of many chronic diseases including cancer.

Financial barriers limit the ability of women, especially the poorest SES group, from utilizing screening and treatment services for early diagnosis and treatment of breast cancer.[2] Increased national commitment to providing breast cancer screening services for all eligible uninsured women has been shown to ultimately reduce morbidity and mortality from breast cancer.[3] Evidence from the United States has shown that prevention, including routine cancer screening, is key to meeting national goals for the elimination of preventable death and suffering due to cancer.[4] Getting the recommended screening tests can be a challenge, particularly with breast cancer and particularly because many women with early breast cancer have no symptoms. There are several screening options required for the diagnosis. The first step in the diagnosis is medical history and BSE. It is vital that women in developing country are educated on how to carry out a breast self examination for any lumps, and when to seek a CBE. Disparities in use of cancer testing are related to differences in income, insurance, race, or ethnicity.[5] A large body of literature has clearly established that economic variables such as health insurance and income affect the receipt of health care services, including cancer screening.[6] Without coverage, women may forgo needed medical services, including screening: uninsured women are 40% less likely to have had a recent mammogram, 26% less likely to have completed a clinical breast examination.[7] Poverty, ignorance and lack of suboptimal health facilities limit the access to screening among Nigerian women.[8]

The next line of action in breast cancer diagnosis is the use of imaging tests such as x-rays. Imaging tests can be used to further study a suspected lump or area of the breast to find out if the suspected lump is cancerous. A mammogram is an x-ray of the breast. Screening mammograms are used to look for breast disease in women who have no signs or symptoms. If abnormalities are present (lump, nipple discharge), a biopsy will be required to determine if it is cancer. BSE, CBE and mammography are the most commonly known and used breast cancer screening methods in the world.[9] Mammography is the most effective screening method for the early detection of breast cancer and it is widely available to women particularly those in the developed world.[10] Uptake in Nigeria is however low because of poor access and unaffordability,[11] but the practice may be low in Nigeria and other developing countries due to cost.[12] Although universal mammography has been shown to result in over diagnosis,[13] the United States Preventive Services Task Force (USPSTF)[14] recommends biennial screening for women 50. The American Cancer Society (ACS)[15] recommends that women 40 and older have a mammogram annually. In Canada and Sweden, there is a 30% mortality reduction from screening women 40 years and older.[16] The American College of Radiology recommends annual screening starting at 40 particularly for women willing to attend follow-up interventions and possible treatment for breast cancer if diagnosed.[17] Mammography is less sensitive and specific particularly among pregnant, premenopausal women and women with dense breast. There is often increased breast density and intense breast cellular proliferative activity during pregnancy as well as the challenge of potentially exposing the developing foetus to radiation.[18] Also benign micro calcifications are common in pregnancy and may give false positive mammography results.[19]

Breast ultrasound or *sonography* can also be used in conjunction with mammography to distinguish between cysts and solid masses. It can potentially be used to differentiate between benign and cancerous tumors. Ultrasonography is usually used in conjunction with mammography, especially when the mammography findings are equivocal. Another potential advantage is that this test is often painless and does not expose the patient to radiation. CBE and breast ultrasonography can also be a good diagnostic tool and should be done in women with high risk of breast cancer.[8] Previous comparative study on the sensitivity of breast sonography, mammography, and clinical breast examination (CBE) indicated that breast sonography had the highest sensitivity.[20] High risk patients or those with dense breast tissue may benefit from additional screening examinations with ultrasound.[21]

Magnetic resonance imaging (MRI) of the breast use radio waves and strong magnets. It is often used along with mammograms for screening women who have a high risk of developing breast cancer. MRI gives a better picture of any suspicious areas found by a mammogram. MRI can also give useful information (actual size of the cancer) in patients with breast cancer. MRI is more accurate than mammography and can accurately detect residual tumour after neoadjuvant chemotherapy.[22] MRI improves sensitivity and is cost-effective for women with BRCA1 and other familial risk for breast cancer, but is expensive, especially in the youngest age categories.[23] Annual screening with MRI is cost-effective for women aged 30 to 60 years with a *BRCA1* or *BRCA2* gene mutation, or women who have a 50% chance of being a carrier.[24] MRI screening is recommended by the United Kingdom's National Institute for Health and Care Excellence (NICE) guideline, the European guideline of the European Society of breast imaging, the American College of Radiologists and American Cancer Society.[25-28] Access to MRI services in Nigeria is significantly low. The limited number who have access to breast cancer screening are universally offered mammography despite not being the ideal screening method; particularly younger women and those with dense breast tissue coupled with the finding that repeated exposure to mammography increases the risk of breast cancer, independent of other factors.[29-30]

Other tests including nipple discharge examined for presence of cancer cells, or red-brown secretions may be suggestive of the presence of blood and a high risk for breast cancer is not present. Biopsy is often carried out when mammograms or other indications show an abnormality that is possibly cancer. During a biopsy, a sample of the suspicious area is removed to be looked at under a microscope. There are several types of biopsies, such as fine needle aspiration biopsy, core (large needle) biopsy, and surgical biopsy. In a fine needle aspiration (FNA) biopsy, a thin, hollow needle is attached to a syringe to withdraw (aspirate) a small amount of tissue from a suspicious area of the breast which is then looked at under a microscope. A core biopsy uses a larger needle to sample breast changes felt by the doctor or pinpointed by ultrasound or mammogram. Also the entire mass or abnormal area, as well as a surrounding margin of normal appearing breast tissue can be removed surgically (excisional biopsy). Lymph node biopsy can also play a role in breast cancer diagnosis, particularly if the lymph nodes under the arm are enlarged which may be checked for cancer spread. In most developed countries, medical care is personalized with each patient being offered the best possible care and treatment based on their individual peculiarities and based on scientific evidence.[31-32] A significant number of women in Nigeria and other countries may not benefit from evidenced- based best practice for a long time. This is an ethical issue of grave public health significance that needs to be addressed.

References

1. Sankaranarayanan R. Screening for cancer in low- and middle-income countries. Ann Glob Health. 2014 Sep-Oct;80(5):412-417.

2. Okoronkwo IL, Ejike-Okoye P, Chinweuba AU, Nwaneri AC. Financial barriers to utilization of screening and treatment services for breast cancer: an equity analysis in Nigeria. Niger J Clin Pract. 2015;18(2):287-291.

3. Lawson HW, Henson R, Bobo JK, Kaeser MK. Implementing recommendations for the early detection of breast and cervical cancer among low-income women. MMWR Recomm Rep. 2000 Mar 31;49(RR-2):37-55.

4. Adams EK, Breen N, Joski PJ. Impact of the National Breast and Cervical Cancer Early Detection Program on mammography and Pap test utilization among white, Hispanic, and African American women: 1996-2000. Cancer. 2007 Jan 15;109(2 Suppl):348-358.

5. Hiatt RA, Klabunde C, Breen N, Swan J, Ballard-Barbash R. Cancer screening practices from National Health Interview Surveys: Past, present, and future. *J Natl Cancer Inst.* 2002; **94**: 1837–1846.

6. Lillie-Blanton M, Hoffman C. The role of health insurance coverage in reducing racial/ethnic disparities in health care. *Health Aff (Millwood). 2005;* **24**: *398–408.*

7. *Fronstin P.* The working uninsured: Who they are, how they have changed, and the consequences of being uninsured—With presidential candidate proposals outlined. EBRI Issue Brief. *2000; 1–23.*

8. Ezeonu Paul Olisaemeka, Ajah Leonard Ogbonna, Onoh Robinson Chukwudi, Lawani Lucky Osaheni, Enemuo Vincent Chidi, Agwu Uzoma MaryRose . Evaluation of clinical breast examination and breast ultrasonography among pregnant women in Abakaliki, Nigeria. Onco Targets Ther. 2015; 8: 1025–1029.

9. Abdel-Fattah M, Zaki A, Bassili A, el-Shazly M, Tognoni G. Breast self-examination practice and its impact on breast cancer diagnosis in Alexandria, Egypt. East Mediterr Health J. 2000 Jan;6(1):34-40

10. Islam SR, Aziz SM. Mammography is the most effective method of breast cancer screening. Mymensingh Med J 2012;21:366-71.

11. Onwere S, Okoro O, Chigbu B, Aluka C, Kamanu C, Onwere A. Breast self-examination as a method of early detection of breast cancer: Knowledge and practice among antenatal clinic attendees in South Eastern Nigeria. Pak J Med Sci 2009;25:122-125.

12. Egwuonwu O A, Anyanwu S, Nwofor A. Default from neoadjuvant chemotherapy in premenopausal female breast cancer patients: What is to blame? Niger J Clin Pract 2012; 15:265-269.

13. Duffy S., Lynge E., Jonsson H, et al. Complexities in the estimation of over diagnosis in breast cancer screening. Br J Cancer 2008;99:1176–1178.

14. U.S. Preventive Services Task Force. Final Update Summary: Breast Cancer: Screening. July 2015

15. American Cancer Society. American Cancer Society Guidelines for the Early Detection of Cancer. March 2015

16. Feig S. Screening mammography benefit controversies: sorting the evidence. Radiol Clin North Am 2014;52:455—480

17. Lee C., Dershaw D., Kopans D, et al. Breast cancer screening with imaging: recommendations from the Society of Breast Imaging and the ACR on the use of mammography, breast MRI, breast ultrasound, and other technologies for the detection of clinically occult breast cancer. J Am Coll Radiol 2010;7:18–27.

18. Buist DS, Porter PL, Lehman C, Taplin SH, White E. Factors contributing to mammography failure in women aged 40–49 years. J Natl Cancer Inst. 2004;96:1432–1440.

19. Stucker DT, Ikeda DM, Hartman AR, et al. New bilateral microcalcifications at mammography in a postlactational woman: case report. Radiology. 2000;217:247–250.

20. Sim L, Hendriks J, Fook-Chong S. Breast ultrasound in women with familial risk of breast cancer. Ann Acad Med Singapore. 2004 Sep;33(5):600-6.

21. Lourenco AP, Mainiero MB. Incorporating Imaging Into the Locoregional Management of Breast Cancer. Semin Radiat Oncol. 2016 Jan;26(1):17-24.

22. Marinovich ML, Houssami N, Macaskill P, Sardanelli F, Irwig L, Mamounas EP, von Minckwitz G, Brennan ME, Ciatto S. Meta-analysis of magnetic resonance imaging in detecting residual breast cancer after neoadjuvant therapy. J Natl Cancer Inst. 2013 Mar 6;105(5):321-333.

23. Saadatmand S, Tilanus-Linthorst MM, Rutgers EJ, Hoogerbrugge N, Oosterwijk JC, Tollenaar RA, Hooning M, Loo CE, Obdeijn IM, Heijnsdijk EA, de Koning HJ. Cost-effectiveness of screening women with familial risk for breast cancer with magnetic resonance imaging. J Natl Cancer Inst. 2013 Sep 4;105(17):1314-21.

24. Lowry KP, Lee JM, Kong CY, McMahon PM, Gilmore ME, Cott Chubiz JE, Pisano ED, Gatsonis C, Ryan PD, Ozanne EM, Gazelle GS. Annual screening strategies in BRCA1 and BRCA2 gene mutation carriers: a comparative effectiveness analysis. Cancer. 2012 Apr 15;118(8):2021-2030.

25. National Institute for Health and Clinical Excellence (NICE). *Familial Breast Cancer: Classification and care of people at risk of familial breast cancer and management of breast cancer and related risks in people with a family history of breast cancer.* NICE Clinical Guideline 164.

26. Mann RM, Kuhl CK, Kinkel K, et al. Breast MRI: guidelines from the European Society of Breast Imaging. *Eur Radiol.* 2008;18(7):1307–1318.

27. American College of Radiology (ACR). *ACR Practice Guideline for the Performance of Contrast enhanced Magnetic Resonance Imaging (MRI) of the Breast.*

28. Saslow D, Boetes C, Burke W, et al. American Cancer Society guidelines for breast screening with MRI as an adjunct to mammography. *CA Cancer J Clin.* 2007;57(2):75–89.

29. Boyd NF, Guo H, Martin LJ, et al. Mammographic density and the risk and detection of breast cancer. *N Engl J Med.* 2007;356(3):227–236.

30. Kerlikowske K. The mammogram that cried Wolfe. *N Engl J Med.* 2007;356(3):297–300.

31. Marino N, Woditschka SL, Reed T, Nakayama J, Mayer M, Wetzel M, Steeg PS. Breast Cancer Metastasis: Issues for the Personalization

of Its Prevention and Treatment. Am J Pathol. 2013 October; 183(4): 1084–1095.

32. Sabatier R, Gonçalves A, Bertucci F. Personalized medicine: present and future of breast cancer management. Crit Rev Oncol Hematol. 2014 Sep;91(3):223-33.

Chapter 6

Late stage breast cancer among premenopausal Nigerian women

The stage at which breast cancer is diagnosed has a tremendous impact on type of treatment, recovery and survival. In most cases, the earlier the cancer is detected and treated the higher the survival rate for the patient. Late presentation of patients at advanced stages when little or no benefit can be derived from any form of therapy is the hallmark of breast cancer in Nigerian women. The mean age at diagnosis of breast cancer in Nigeria was 42.7 years (SD 12.2, range 18-85 years). Patients less than 40 years accounted for 39.8% of the total number of patients with infiltrating breast carcinoma.[1] Breast cancer is now the commonest malignancy affecting women in Nigeria.[2] It is likely to become an important public health issue in coming years.[3] Diagnostic and treatment delays in Nigerian seem to be responsible for the high prevalence of more advanced and higher grade (stage 3 and 4) breast cancer in Nigeria. Nigerian breast cancers are often high-grade, late-stage, high-proliferating and occur in a younger population than those of the Western countries.[1] In Nigeria, the mean age at presentation of breast cancer is low compared to observation in the developed world. A significant number of cases of breast cancer among women of African descent are the more advanced stages 3 and 4. A previous report compared the histology and patterns of occurrence of breast cancers in Nigeria (n = 297) and Finland (n = 285). The mean age at presentation was 42.7 years in Nigeria versus 58.7 years in Finland. In both populations there was an association between reproductive factors and the occurrence of breast cancer. In Nigeria, 53.2% of cases belonged to stages 3 and 4, versus 6.7% in Finland. In Finland there were higher frequencies of lobular, tubular and mucinous types than in Nigeria. The Nigerian material had more medullary type (2.7% vs. 0.7% in Finland), extensive necrosis, nuclear atypia and pleomorphism, with coexisting pleomorphic ductal carcinoma in situ. At 2 years after treatment, the survival figures for Nigeria and Finland were 72.8% and 96.4%, respectively.[1] Early detection through the use of mammography, high-quality surgery, and adjuvant therapies including chemotherapy and targeted therapies, such as hormonal therapy and, more recently the HER2-directed agent trastuzumab, can be credited for much of the recent improvement in outcome for women with breast cancer in the USA.[4] Experience about breast cancer in Eastern, Midwestern, Western Nigeria, South Eastern Nigeria and the Niger Delta of Nigeria respectively shows that it follows a pattern similar to other parts of the developed world except that many present late in mainly multiparous pre-menopausal and low income patients. [5-10] Late presentation has a number of implications. It is often associated with aggressive features, poor survival and a high chance of occurrence of presenting to emergency unit as an oncologic emergency. A previous report to evaluate the pattern of oncologic emergencies seen in adult cancer patients in Ahmadu Bello University Teaching Hospital, Zaria, Nigeria indicated that tumour haemorrhage is the commonest oncologic emergency commonly seen in metastatic and locally advanced disease in Nigeria.[11] The skeleton is the commonest site of metastases from breast carcinoma. Radionuclide isotope scanning is a sensitive scanning procedure for the demonstration of bone pathology. Previous report indicate that there is scintigraphic evidence of bone metastasis in most patients with stage four breast cancers, and in some with locally advanced disease. Multiple bone lesions are commonly found in women with advanced breast cancer in Nigeria and almost all the lesions were osteoblastic involving both the truncal and axial skeletal bones.[12] A previous study to describe the frequency, stages, histological patterns, staging and grading of BRCA in a local scenario of a tertiary hospital in southern Nigeria indicated that late presentation (Stages III and IV) constituted 76.2% of breast cancer.[8] This finding is similar to reports of other researchers[13-14] who reported 67% and 64% respectively. Also, Adesunkanmi and colleagues[15] observed that 74% of BRCA present in Stages III and IV. The reason for the late presentation in Nigeria is partly attributable to poverty and ignorance. Previous report has shown that women with breast cancer living in areas with limited access to healthcare services are more likely to have been diagnosed with late stage breast cancer.[16] A retrospective study carried out to examine five year survival from breast cancer cases diagnosed between 2005 and May

2008 in Nigerian women revealed that the different staging of disease and treatment are independent predictors of disease outcome, whereas age of diagnosis and menopausal status although associated with low hazards are not significant. The study observed a five year breast cancer survival rate in Lagos, Nigeria of 24.1% (54/224). Poor survival rates are mainly attributed to late presentation and poor follow-up, hence early detection through breast cancer awareness programs, appropriate logistics and better management of patients through guidelines for the treatment of breast cancer need to be implemented to improve survival.[17] According to the International Agency for Research on Cancer, breast cancer is the most frequently diagnosed cancer among women, with an estimated 1.38 million cases diagnosed worldwide in 2008. It is also the most frequently reported cause of death from cancer in women in both developed and developing countries.

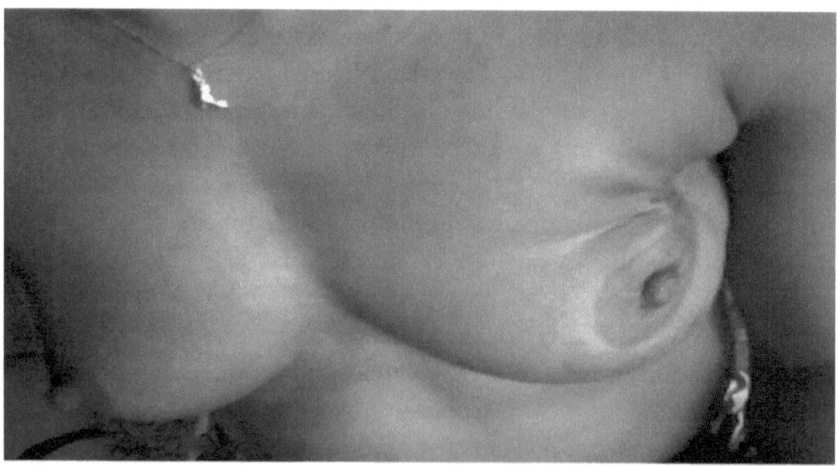

Figure 5: Advanced breast cancer in a 31 years old Nigerian woman

Table 1: Breast Cancer Survival Rate depending on state stage of diagnosis and management

Stage of Breast Cancer	Survival Rate
Stage 0	100%
Stage I	98%
Stage II	56%
Stage IIIA	49%
Stage IV	16%

Breast cancer survival rates vary greatly worldwide, ranging from 80% or more in North America, Sweden and Japan to about 60% in middle income countries, and less than 40% in low income countries. The low survival rates in less developed countries are mainly due to late diagnosis of the majority of cases. The Nigerian health system is all there is for a significant number of Nigerians who cannot afford to go on medical tourism to India or other developed countries. The Nigerian nation has health professionals with the skill required for the effective management of women with breast cancer, and the professionals are willing and committed to delivering better healthcare service. They are however constrained by the lack of an enabling environment, poor infrastructure and poor remuneration. African American women (AAW) are 25% more likely to present with late stage breast cancer, and 20% more likely to die from their disease than Caucasian women. Socioeconomic factors, lack of access and knowledge, spiritual and religious beliefs, fear and fatalism are reported as contributing factors to screening delays.[18] It needs to be noted however that AAW diagnosed at age 57 or more have superior breast cancer outcome compared to white US women also of that age group.[19-20] Thus there is apparently a racial disparity inversion at age 57 so we need to consider biology as a racial disparity factor. Women who were less educated, unmarried, and talked to God only about their breast change were significantly more likely to delay seeking medical care. An association was found between disclosing a breast symptom to God only, and delay in seeking medical care. In contrast, women who had told a person about their breast symptom were more likely to seek medical care sooner.[21] Previous study has advocated that for breast cancer prevention programs in Nigeria to succeed, they must in addition to breast awareness and screening programs, address the institutional bottlenecks, the dearth of knowledge among primary care physicians and improve referrals from alternative practitioners and prayer houses.[22-23] Financial barriers limit the ability of women, especially those in the poorest socioeconomic group, to utilize screening and treatment services for early diagnosis and treatment of breast cancer. Interventions that will improve financial risk protection for women with breast cancer or at risk of breast cancer are needed to ensure equitable access to screening and treatment services.[24-25] Delayed treatment of symptomatic breast cancer in Nigeria is as much related to the quality of medical care, local beliefs, ignorance of the disease, and lack of acceptance of orthodox treatment.[26]

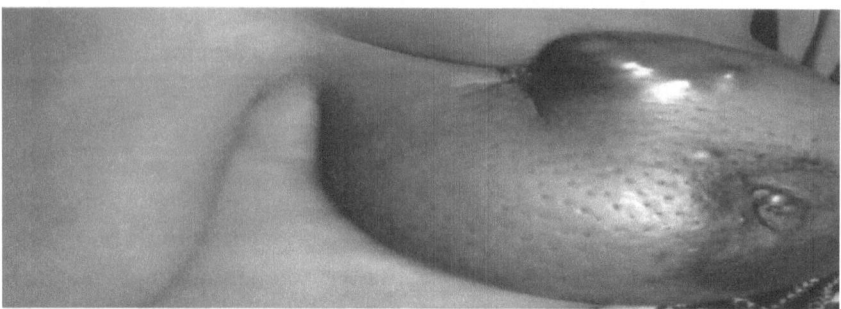

Figure 6: Stage 4 Breast Cancer in a Nigerian Woman

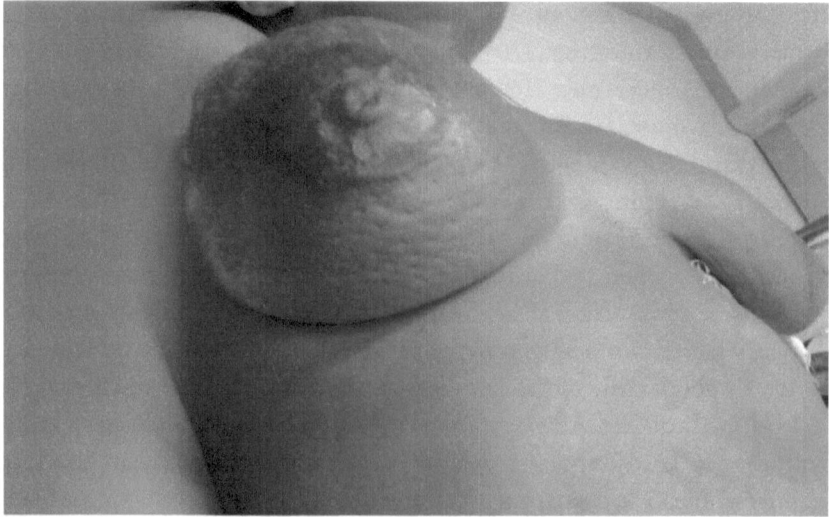

Figure 7: Right Inflammatory Breast Cancer in a Nigerian Woman

*Breast Cancer in Nigeria:
Diagnosis, Management and Challenges*

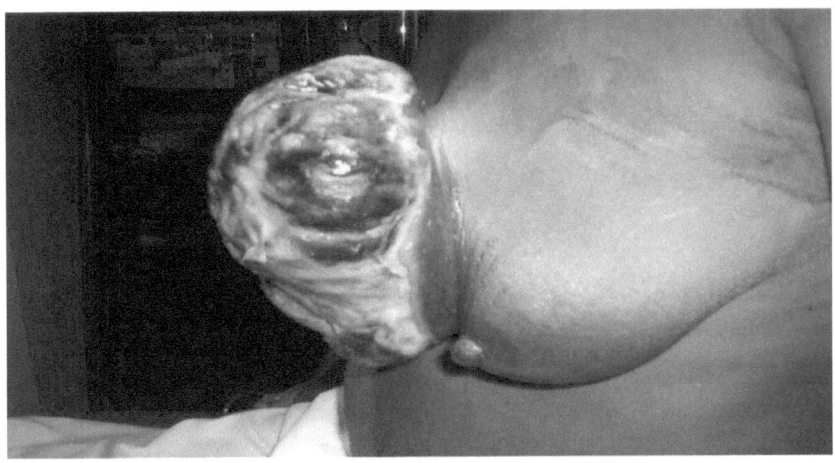

Figure 8: Advanced stage breast cancer in a Nigerian woman

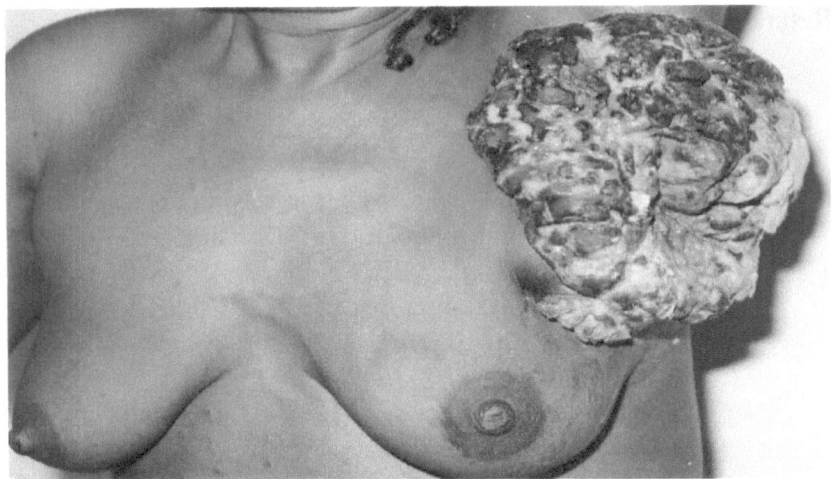

Figure 9: Stage 4 Breast Cancer in a Nigerian woman

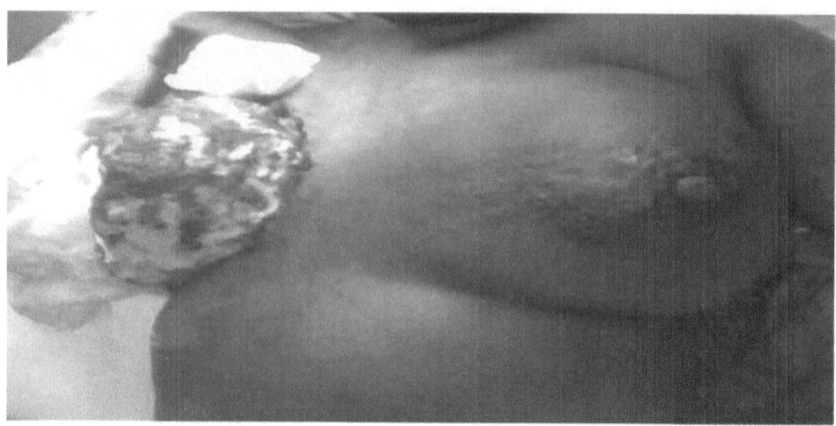

Figure 10: Stage 4 breast cancer in a Nigerian woman

References

1. Ikpat OF, Ndoma-Egba R, Collan Y. Influence of age and prognosis of breast cancer in Nigeria. East Afr Med J. 2002; 79(12):651-657.

2. Adebamowo CA. Cancer incidence in Nigeria: a report from population-based cancer registries. Cancer Epidemiol. 2012; 36(5):e271-278.

3. Afolayan EA. Five years of Cancer Registration at Zaria (1992 - 1996). Niger *Postgrad Med J.* 2004; 11(3):225-229.

4. Sloan FA, Gelband H, editors. *Cancer Control Opportunities in Low- and Middle-Income Countries.* Washington, DC, USA: Institute of Medicine of the National Academies; 2007.

5. Anyanwu SN. Breast cancer in eastern Nigeria: a ten year review. West Afr J Med 2000; 19(2):120-125.

6. Abudu EK, Banjo AA, Izegbu MC, Agboola AO, Anunobi CC, Musa OA. (2007). Malignant Breast Lessons at Olabisi Onabanjo University Teaching Hospital (O.O.U.T.H), Sagamu-a Histopathological Review. Niger Postgraduate Medical Journal; 14(1):57-59.

7. Ekanem VJ, Aligbe JU.Histopathological types of breast cancer in Nigerian women: a 12-year review (1993-2004). Afr J Reprod Health. 2006;10(1):71-75.

8. Forae G, Nwachokor F, Igbe A. Histopathological profile of breast cancer in an African population. Ann Med Health Sci Res. 2014; 4(3):369-373.

9. Ntekim A, Nufu FT, Campbell OB. Breast cancer in young women in Ibadan, Nigeria. Afr Health Sci. 2009; 9(4):242-246.

10. Njeze GE. Breast lumps: a 21-year single-center clinical and histological analysis. Niger J Surg. 2014 ;20(1):38-41.

11. Adewuyi SA, Ajekigbe AT, Campbell OB, Mbibu NH, Oguntayo AO, Kolawole AO, et al. Pattern of oncologic emergencies seen in adult cancer patients attending the Radiotherapy and Oncology Centre, Ahmadu Bello University Teaching Hospital, Zaria - Nigeria. *Niger Postgrad Med J*. 2012; 19(4):208-214.

12. Ogundiran TO, Ayandipo OO, Adedapo KS, Orunmuyi AT, Ademola AF, Onimode YA, Ayeni OA, Alonge TO. Bone Scintigraphy in Breast Cancer Patients in Ibadan, Nigeria. West Afr J Med. 2014; 33(3):172-177.

13. Anyanwu SN, Egwuonwu OA, Ihekwoaba EC. Acceptance and adherence to treatment among breast cancer patients in Eastern Nigeria. Breast. 2011; 20 (2):S51-53.

14. Osime CO, Dongo AE. Presentation, pattern and outcome of breast cancer in a poor economy: A definition of the tripod of ignorance, disease and poverty. Emerg Med J. 2012; 11:20–28.

15. Adesunkanmi AR, Lawal OO, Adelusola KA, Durosimi MA. The severity, outcome and challenges of breast cancer in Nigeria. *Breast*. 2006; 15:399–409.

16. Williams F, Jeanetta S, O'Brien DJ, Fresen JL. Rural-urban difference in female breast cancer diagnosis in Missouri. Rural Remote Health. 2015; 15(3):3063.

17. Makanjuola SB, Popoola AO, Oludara MA. Radiation therapy: a major factor in the five-year survival analysis of women with breast cancer in Lagos, Nigeria. Radiother Oncol. 2014;111(2):321-326.

18. Gullate M. The influence of spirituality and religiosity on breast cancer screening delay in African American women: application of the Theory of Reasoned Action and Planned Behavior (TRA/TPB). ABNF J. 2006 Spring; 17(2):89-94.

19. Retsky MW, Demicheli R, Gukas ID, Hrushesky WJ. Enhanced surgery-induced angiogenesis among premenopausal women might partially explain excess breast cancer mortality of blacks compared to whites: an hypothesis. Int J Surg. 2007 Oct;5(5):300-3004.

20. Demicheli R, Retsky MW, Hrushesky WJ, Baum M, Gukas ID, Jatoi I. Racial disparities in breast cancer outcome: insights into host-tumor interactions. Cancer. 2007 Nov 1;110(9):1880-8. Review.

21. Gullatte MM, Brawley O, Kinney A, Powe B, Mooney K. Religiosity, spirituality, and cancer fatalism beliefs on delay in breast cancer diagnosis in African American women. J Relig Health. 2010; 49(1):62-72.

22. Ezeome ER. Delays in presentation and treatment of breast cancer in Enugu, Nigeria. Niger J Clin Pract. 2010; 13(3):311-316.

23. Kene TS, Odigie VI, Yusufu LM, Yusuf BO, Shehu SM, Kase JT. Pattern of presentation and survival of breast cancer in a teaching hospital in north Western Nigeria. Oman Med J. 2010; 25(2):104-107.

24. Ali R, Mathew A, Rajan B. Effects of socio-economic and demographic factors in delayed reporting and late-stage presentation among patients with breast cancer in a major cancer hospital in South India. *Asian Pac J Cancer Prev.* 2008; 9(4):703-707.

25. Okoronkwo IL, Ejike-Okoye P, Chinweuba AU, Nwaneri AC. Financial barriers to utilization of screening and treatment services

for breast cancer: an equity analysis in Nigeria. Niger J Clin Pract. 2015;18(2):287-291.

26. Ukwenya AY, Yusufu LM, Nmadu PT, Garba ES, Ahmed A. Delayed treatment of symptomatic breast cancer: the experience from Kaduna, Nigeria. S Afr J Surg. 2008; 46(4):106-110.

Chapter 7

Challenge of Triple Negative Brest Cancer (TNBC) in Nigeria

Triple negative breast cancer (TNBC) refers to any breast cancer that does not express the genes for oestrogen receptor (ER), progesterone receptor (PR) or Her2/neu. With immunohistochemistry (IHC), breast cancer is classified into four groups based on IHC profile of oestrogen receptor (ER)/progesterone receptor (PR) and human epidermal growth factor receptor 2 (HER2/neu) expression, positive (+) and/or negative (-). The IHC classification correlates well with intrinsic gene expression microarray categorization. ER positive tumours may benefit from being treated with selective ER modulators and aromatase inhibitors, whereas patients with HER2/neu positive tumours have been shown to experience a significant survival advantage when treated with humanized monoclonal antibodies against HER2/neu. This makes it more difficult to treat TNBC since most chemotherapeutic agents target one of the three receptors. Triple negative breast cancers have a relapse pattern that is very different from hormone positive breast cancers: the risk of relapse is much higher for the first 3–5 years but drops sharply and substantially below that of hormone positive breast cancers.[1-2] Triple negative breast cancer tends to be very aggressive, metastasizes soon after therapy. The results of combination therapy trials for TNBC are somewhat promising, although more effective treatments are still needed. Trials of different combination therapies are ongoing, so patients with TNBC should consider enrolling in trials and should always discuss all their treatment options with their doctors. Patients with TNBC tend to have worse clinical outcomes as a result of lacking a therapeutic target. About three quarters of triple negative breast cancers (TNBCs) are estrogen receptor (ER) negative, progesterone receptor (PR) negative and do not over express HER2.[3] For 30 years, accumulating evidence suggests that obese women have poorer prognoses than lean ones after breast cancer treatment.[4-5] In an observational prospective study of about 350,000 US women, higher BMI was very significantly associated with increasing risk of dying from breast cancer.[6] The typical type of breast cancer in Nigeria is triple negative (TNBC) and as noted is usually considered the worst early breast cancer diagnosis, since there are no known targeted therapies and patients often relapse and die early. Expression of oestrogen receptors (ER) and progesterone receptors (PR) and Human Epidermal Growth Factor Receptor (HER-2) in breast carcinomas identifies patients that are more likely to respond to targeted adjuvant therapy. Breast cancer is the most common cancer among women globally. Triple negative breast cancers are common in Nigeria (29.2%), and affect young females and could be contributory to the poorer prognosis of breast cancer in our environment.[7] These findings underscore the urgent need for research into the aetiology and treatment of the aggressive molecular subtypes that disproportionately affect young women of African descent. A previous report among breast cancer subjects in Calabar, Nigeria indicated that ER and PR were immunohistochemically detected in 24.0% and 13.9%, respectively.[8] A previous report among Nigeria women with breast cancer in Abia State, Nigeria indicated that the majority of cases were high grade (100% were grade III), triple-negative (65%), and occur in young women (mean age 47 years).[9] Several studies have suggested that breast cancer in Black women is associated with aggressive features and poor survival. A previous report in Jos, Nigeria examined molecular markers along with clinical stage and pathological grade in breast cancer. Results indicated that there is predominance of high grade, invasive ductal carcinomas which are likely to be ER and PGR negative but p53 positive. These features suggest a biologically aggressive form of breast cancer in Nigerian women with the possibility of poor response to both hormonal therapy and chemotherapy.[10] Similarly, a study has reported that the prevalence of ER negative tumours in breast cancer patients is much higher in black women than in white women in the US. The prevalence of ER negative tumours significantly varied from 22.0 % (n = 41/186) in Eastern Africans to 32.9 % (n = 47/143) in Western African Blacks. The prevalence was similar in West African born and Jamaican born Blacks, but significantly lower in East African born Blacks. Notably, the ER negative prevalence in East African born Blacks was comparable to the US born Whites with breast cancer.[11] Also, a study involving 507 patients diagnosed with breast cancer between 1996 and 2007 at six geographic regions in Nigeria and Senegal indicated that compared with White women, Black women experience a disproportionate burden of aggressive breast cancer. Triple negativity for HER-2, ER and PR markers was predominant, including basal-like (27%) and unclassified subtype (28%). Other subtypes were luminal A (27%), luminal B (2%), and HER2 positive/ER negative (15%).[12] A study to determine the prevalence of oestrogen and progesterone receptor positivity among histologically diagnosed breast cancer cases at the University of Benin Teaching Hospital, Benin City, Nigeria indicated a steroid hormone receptor positivity of 17%. Oestrogen and progesterone receptor positivity were 14.1% and 9.6% respectively.[13] Advances in breast cancer research have demonstrated differences between Black and White women regarding tumour behaviour, patient outcome and response to treatment. The tumour suppressor gene p53 has been speculated to be involved in tumour biology of triple negative and/or basal-like BC, and more commonly observed in Black than Caucasian women. Targeting the p53 pathways for therapeutic usage might improve the poor outcome observed among Nigerian women. A previous report investigated the protein expression of p53 in tissue samples from a series of 308 Nigerian women. Clinicopathological parameters, biomarkers of functional significance in breast cancer and patient outcome of tumours expressing p53 in Nigerian women were correlated with UK grade matched series. A significantly large proportion of BC from Nigerian women showed high p53 expression compared with UK women. In those tumours showing positive p53 in the Nigerian series, a significant proportion were premenopausal, diagnosed before 50 years, larger in size, with evidence of metastasis into lymphatic vessels. In addition, p53 positive expression was also significantly correlated with negative expression of ER and PgR, BRCA1, MDM2, p21 and E-cadherin and positively associated with P-cadherin, triple negative phenotype, basal cytokeratin (CK) 5/6 expression and basal phenotype compared with the UK series. Survival analyses showed that Nigerian women with breast cancer were significantly associated with poor breast cancer specific survival, but no significant association with disease free interval was observed.[14] Triple negative breast cancers are common in Nigeria, and affect young females and contribute to the poorer prognosis of breast cancer in Nigeria. A previous report in Lagos, Nigeria to determine ER/PR, HER2/neu expression and their association with histological prognostic markers in female breast carcinomas indicated that about 18.7% of breast cancers had IHC (ER, PR and HER2) done.

IHC pattern was as follows: ER/PR+, HER2- = 19 (39.6%), ER/PR-, HER2- (triple negative [TN]) = 14 (29.2%), ER/PR+, HER2+ = 9 (18.8%), ER/PR-, HER2+ = 6 (12.5%), corresponding to Lumina A, TN/basal-like, Lumina B and HER2 over expressed respectively.[15] A British study also found that Black women presented at a younger age with a higher frequency of grade 3, ER-negative tumors and had poorer outcomes than white patients with breast cancer.[16]

Epidemiologic evidence suggests that Korean women have a lower incidence of breast cancer than women in the United States. Patients in US were more likely to have hormone receptor positive breast cancer, while patients in Republic of Korea have a higher rate of triple negative lesions.[17] As it is among Nigerian women and Korean women, breast cancer in African Americans is more likely to be early onset, higher grade, and estrogen receptor (ER) negative compared with breast cancer in white Americans.[18-20]

A previous study involving 500 patients with breast cancer from different geographic regions in West Africa, found that hormone receptor negative breast cancer is predominant, and only 25% were ER positive. Previous report in Nigeria reported 25%, 24% and 71% ER positive respectively.[8, 10, 21] The proportion of ER positive breast cancer in Blacks living in the United States and United Kingdom has been consistently reported between 61% and 66%.[16,18] Compared with White women, Black women experience a disproportionate burden of aggressive breast cancer for reasons that remain unknown and understudied. A previous study that investigated the distribution of molecular subtypes of invasive breast tumors in indigenous Black women in West Africa indicated that the proportions of estrogen receptor (ER) positive, progesterone receptor positive, and human epidermal growth factor receptor 2 (HER2) positive tumors were 24%, 20%, and 17%, respectively. Triple negativity for these markers was predominant, including basal like (27%) and unclassified subtype (28%). Other subtypes were luminal A (27%), luminal B (2%), and HER2 positive/ER negative (15%).[12]

Triple negative breast cancers (TNBCs) represent a distinct subgroup of breast cancers with an immunohistochemical phenotype that is negative for oestrogen receptor (ER), progesterone receptor (PR), and human epidermal growth factor receptor 2 (HER-2).[22] Triple negative breast cancers doesn't respond to many standard breast cancer treatments, but clinical trials of combination therapies are showing possible promise. Although breast cancer survival rates are improving on the whole, those for women diagnosed with the triple-negative form remain significantly lower. Largely, that is because triple-negative breast cancer (TNBC) do not respond to many of the more modern, targeted treatments. Breast cancer in India is the second commonest cancer in females there. In a previous report, triple-negative breast cancers constituted 22.7% of cases among South Indian breast cancer patients.[23] Similarly, a previous report that examined the incidence of breast cancer with triple-negative phenotype (TNBC) in a cohort of 499 patients without distant metastases indicated that three hundred and thirty subjects (66.2%) had triple-negative breast cancer; defined as those that had "negative" level of oestrogen and progesterone receptors and were HER2neu negative.[24] A study among 149 Brazilian women indicated that oestrogen receptor (ER) was positive in 59.6% cases, HER2 overexpression was detected in 32.8%, a low prevalence of Luminal A and a high prevalence of triple negative cases.[25]

Triple-negative breast cancer (TNBC) is known to be associated with aggressive biologic features and a poor clinical outcome. Therefore, early detection of TNBC with few false negatives is considered mandatory to improve prognosis.[26] Advances in understanding tumour biology, particularly signalling pathways, have led to the development and approval of many novel agents and have changed the landscape of therapy for patients with metastatic breast cancer. While significant progress has been made in treating certain types of breast cancer, triple-negative metastatic breast cancer unfortunately remains especially challenging.[27] For patients with metastatic breast cancer, expanding therapeutic options through clinical trial participation is a crucial part of modern oncology practice. Several strategies have been implemented to overcome endocrine and human epidermal growth factor 2-neu (HER2) resistance, targeting triple-negative breast cancers (which do not express the HER2, oestrogen, and progesterone receptors) through novel receptors, harnessing the immune system, and new ways of targeting angiogenesis.[28] CXCR4 may be an effective target for nanocarrier-based therapies particularly in TNBC. CXCR4 is a cell membrane receptor that is overexpressed in triple-negative breast cancers and implicated in growth and metastasis of this disease. Targeted nanocarriers are selectively taken up by CXCR4-expressing cells and effectively block CXCR4 signalling.[29]

References

1. Cheang, M. C. U.; Voduc, D.; Bajdik, C.; Leung, S.; McKinney, S.; Chia, S. K.; Perou, C. M.; Nielsen, T. O. (2008). "Basal-Like Breast Cancer Defined by Five Biomarkers Has Superior Prognostic Value than Triple-Negative Phenotype". Clinical Cancer Research; 14 (5): 1368–1376.

2. Hudis, C. A.; Gianni, L.Triple-Negative Breast Cancer: An Unmet Medical Need". The Oncologist 2011; 16: 1–11.

3. Carey LA, Perou CM, Livasy CA, Dressler LG, Cowan D, Conway K, et al. Race, breast cancer subtypes, and survival in the Carolina Breast Cancer Study. Jama. 2006; 295(21):2492–502.

4. Dawood S, Broglio K, Gonzalez-Angulo AM, Kau SW, Islam R, Hortobagyi GN, et al. Prognostic value of body mass index in locally advanced breast cancer. Clinical cancer research: an official journal of the American Association for Cancer Research. 2008; 14(6):1718–1725.

5. Kroenke CH, Chen WY, Rosner B, Holmes MD. Weight, weight gain, and survival after breast cancer diagnosis. Journal of clinical oncology: official journal of the American Society of Clinical Oncology. 2005; 23(7):1370–1378.

6. Ewertz M, Jensen MB, Gunnarsdottir KA, Hojris I, Jakobsen EH, Nielsen D, et al. Effect of obesity on prognosis after early-stage breast cancer. Journal of clinical oncology: official journal of the American Society of Clinical Oncology. 2011; 29(1):25–31.

7. Nwafor CC, Keshinro SO. Pattern of hormone receptors and human epidermal growth factor receptor 2 status in sub-Saharan breast cancer cases: Private practice experience. J Clin Oncol. 2009 Sep 20; 27(27): 4515–4521.

8. Ikpatt OF, Ndoma-Egba R. Oestrogen and progesterone receptors in Nigerian breast cancer: relationship to tumour histopathology and survival of patients. Cent Afr J Med. 2003; 49(11-12):122-126.

9. Adisa CA, Eleweke N, Alfred AA, Campbell MJ, Sharma R, Nseyo O, Tandon V, Mukhtar R, Greninger A, Risi JD, Esserman LJ. Biology of breast cancer in Nigerian women: a pilot study. *Ann Afr Med*. 2012; 11(3):169-175.

10. Gukas ID, Jennings BA, Mandong BM, et al. Clinicopathological features and molecular markers of breast cancer in Jos, Nigeria. West Afr J Med. 2005; 24:209–213.

11. Jemal A, Fedewa SA. Is the prevalence of ER-negative breast cancer in the US higher among Africa-born than US-born black women? Breast Cancer Res Treat. 2012;135(3):867-873.

12. Huo D, Ikpatt F, Khramtsov A, Dangou JM, Nanda R, Dignam J, Zhang B, Grushko T, Zhang C, Oluwasola O, Malaka D, Malami S, Odetunde A, Adeoye AO, Iyare F, Falusi A, Perou CM, Olopade OI. Population differences in breast cancer: survey in indigenous African women reveals over-representation of triple-negative breast cancer. J Clin Oncol. 2009; 27(27):4515-4521.

13. Ugiagbe EE, Obaseki DE, Oluwasola AO, Olu-Eddo AN, Akhiwu WO. Frequency of distribution of oestrogen and progesterone receptors positivities in breast cancer cases in Benin-City, Nigeria. Niger Postgrad Med J. 2012;19(1):19-24.

14. Agboola AO, Banjo AA, Anunobi CC, Ayoade BA, Deji-Agboola AM, Musa AA, Abdel-Fatah T, Nolan CC, Rakha EA, Ellis IO, Green AR. Molecular profiling of breast cancer in Nigerian women identifies an altered p53 pathway as a major mechanism underlying its poor prognosis compared with British counterpart. *Malays J Pathol*. 2014; 36(1):3-17.

15. Nwafor CC, Keshinro SO.Pattern of hormone receptors and human epidermal growth factor receptor 2 status in sub-Saharan breast cancer cases: Private practice experience. Niger J Clin Pract. 2015; 18(4):553-558.

16. Bowen RL, Duffy SW, Ryan DA, et al. Early onset of breast cancer in a group of British black women. Br J Cancer. 2008; 98:277–281.

17. Son BH, Dominici LS, Aydogan F, Shulman LN, Ahn SH, Cho JY, Coopey SB, Kim SB, Min HE, Valero M, Wang J, Caragacianu D, Gong GY, Hevelone ND, Baek S, Golshan M. Young women with breast cancer in the United States and South Korea: comparison of demographics, pathology and management. Asian Pac J Cancer Prev. 2015; 16(6):2531-2535.

18. Chu KC, Anderson WF. Rates for breast cancer characteristics by estrogen and progesterone receptor status in the major racial/ethnic groups. Breast Cancer Res Treat. 2002; 74:199–211.

19. Eley JW, Hill HA, Chen VW, et al. Racial differences in survival from breast cancer: Results of the National Cancer Institute Black/White Cancer Survival Study. JAMA. 1994; 272:947–954.

20. Smith-Bindman R, Miglioretti DL, Lurie N, et al. Does utilization of screening mammography explain racial and ethnic differences in breast cancer. Ann Intern Med. 2006; 144:541–553.

21. Adebamowo CA, Famooto A, Ogundiran TO, et al. Immunohistochemical and molecular subtypes of breast cancer in Nigeria. Breast Cancer Res Treat 2008; 110: 183–188.

22. Sharma S, Barry M, Gallagher DJ, Kell M, Sacchini V. An overview of triple negative breast cancer for surgical oncologists. Surg Oncol. 2015: S0960-7404(15)30006-32.

23. Patnayak R, Jena A, Rukmangadha N, Chowhan AK, Sambasivaiah K, Phaneendra BV, Reddy MK. Hormone receptor status (estrogen receptor, progesterone receptor), human epidermal growth factor-2 and p53 in South Indian breast cancer patients: A tertiary care center experience. Indian J Med Paediatr Oncol. 2015; 36(2):117-22.

24. Zhukova LG. Breast cancer with triple-negative phenotype in the Russian patient population. Clinical and morphologic features. Vopr Onkol. 2015; 61(2):189-194.

25. de Deus Moura R, Carvalho FM, Bacchi CE. Breast cancer in very young women: Clinicopathological study of 149 patients ≤25 years old. Breast. 2015 ;24(4):461-467.

26. Kim MY, Choi N. Mammographic and ultrasonographic features of triple-negative breast cancer: a comparison with other breast cancer subtypes. Acta Radiol. 2013;54(8):889-894.

27. Campone M, Valo I, Jézéquel P, Moreau M, Boissard A, Campion L, Loussouarn D, Verriele V, Coqueret O, Guette C.Prediction of recurrence and survival for triple-negative breast cancer by a protein signature in tissue samples. Mol Cell Proteomics. 2015 Jul 24. pii: mcp.M115.048967.

28. Santa-Maria CA, Gradishar WJ. Changing Treatment Paradigms in Metastatic Breast Cancer: Lessons Learned. JAMA Oncol. 2015 Jul 1;1(4):528-534.

29. Misra AC, Luker KE, Durmaz H, Luker GD, Lahann J. CXCR4-Targeted Nanocarriers for Triple Negative Breast Cancers. Biomacromolecules. 2015 Jul 22.

Chapter 8

Challenges Associated with Carrying out Randomized Clinical Trials on Breast Cancer in Nigeria

A randomized controlled trial (RCT) is a type of scientific (often medical) experiment, where the people being studied are allocated at random (by chance alone) to receive one of several clinical interventions.[1] The RCT is generally seen as the gold standard for a clinical trial. They are used to test the efficacy or effectiveness of various types of medical intervention with the aim of obtaining evidence- based information about adverse effects and drug reactions. The RCT is one of the simplest and most powerful tools in clinical research. In RCT one of these interventions serve as a standard (control) upon which the comparison with the test `is based. The control may be a standard practice, a placebo or no intervention at all. Individuals in RCT are called a participant or subject. The aim of RCTs is to measure (quantitatively) and compare the outcomes (subjects) and control after the subjects receive the interventions. In sum, RCTs are quantitative, comparative, controlled experiments in which investigators study two or more interventions in a series of individuals who receive them in random order. Peculiarities with RCT is that they are a controlled experiment, have a clinical event as an outcome measure, done in a clinical setting, involves subjects suffering from a specific disease or health condition upon which the trial is based and participants are randomly assigned to different groups that compare different treatments.

Most chemotherapeutic regimens being used for the management of Breast cancer patients in the developing countries have been tested in clinical trials in the developed world, and findings may not be generalizable to the developing world, where patient and tumor characteristics may differ markedly. This is an ethical issue of public health significance. There is growing advocacy and justification to carry out more clinical trials in developing countries to generate evidenced-based information that can facilitate the effect management of women with breast cancer in developing countries. [2]

Breast cancer is a rapidly emerging disease in sub Saharan Africa and affected women tend to be younger, poor and present with late stage disease.[3-5] There are several challenges associated with research governance on breast cancer in Nigeria compared to the developed economies.[6] Ethics approval in Nigeria tend not be as well structured as it is in the West. Tracing patients and follow-up is often difficult. Record keeping and data retrieval have deficiencies. Lack of accurate, supporting databases such as cancer registries,[7] population census, and demography make interpretation of research information difficult. Also the health infrastructures tend to be suboptimal,[8] the people tend to be poor, health tends not to be universal, many patients present to hospital late because they cannot afford cost of diagnosis, surgery and follow-up monitoring. The only way clinical trials on breast cancer can realistically happen in Nigeria is if diagnosis, surgery and post surgical management is done at a no cost implication to the patients. If not, the chance of losing patients to follow-up is high. It is a vital safeguard to plan research, trial or study that takes into consideration these challenges in the planning stages rather than to encounter them midway through the study.[9] Research to develop these new treatments and others, particularly from natural or repurposed products is urgently needed and this can be done safely within established clinical trials with the right health research ethics and regulatory frameworks.[10] There are several challenges associated with carrying out effective randomized clinical trials on breast cancer in Nigeria and other developing countries; follow up challenges, cost challenges, late stage presentation, high prevalence of triple negative breast cancers, suboptimal health infrastructure, lack of governance, suboptimal number of trained clinical trial personnel, poor laboratory capacity, informed consent- related challenges, ethical challenges, poor data management, suboptimal number of trained statisticians, challenge of poor awareness and stigma associated with breast cancer, patronage of traditional healers and spiritualist, dealing with conflict of interest, poor trail design, logistics and accessibility issues associated with the management of health products, education and communication-related challenges, challenge of randomization, cultural and religious issues and bureaucracy in government.[11-23] There is need for funding agencies to step in to solve this ethical issue by massively investing in clinical trials in breast cancer in developing countries. What is desperately need is international collaborations between researchers from developed countries and those from developing economies in carrying out randomized clinical trials aimed at providing evidence-based, resource-stratified guidelines for the management and control of breast cancer. [24] Carrying out meaningful randomized clinical trial on breast cancer in Nigeria and other developing countries is the only way to develop evidence-based, economically feasible, religious and culturally appropriate data for the effective management of breast cancer in developing countries.[25]

One of the ways Nigeria and other developing countries can effectively fight the war against breast cancer is by developing new and affordable treatments through established clinical trials. Surgery is the main modality of local treatment for breast cancer. Surgery and/or radiotherapy can control loco-regional disease in the majority of patients. However, more than 60% of patients will ultimately die due to distant recurrence of disease. Two types of systemic adjuvant therapy have been used increasingly over the last years to successfully reduce the rate of breast cancer recurrence and death. Adjuvant chemotherapy involves a combination of cytotoxic anticancer drugs; adjuvant hormone therapy deprives cancer cells of the hormone oestrogen, which some breast cancer cells need to grow. These therapeutic modalities are complementary and are often used in combination. Most relapses (50–80%) reside in this first peak, while the others are distributed mostly around the third to the sixth postoperative years. The hazard rate of early recurrence is greater in high risk patients (the type commonly seen in Nigeria and other developed countries) identified with worse primary tumour characteristics (large size, high grade and lymph node involvement). Recently, a Belgian group reported data from a retrospective disease free survival study of 327 consecutive patients who were compared according to the perioperative cheap and affordable analgesics administered (sufentanil, clonidine, ketorolac and ketamine. [26] Chemotherapy, radiotherapy and endocrine therapy were performed according to the international expert consensus (9th and 10th St-Gallen consensus). Follow-up in that initial report was average 27.3 months with range 13-44 months. Perioperative administration of the Non-Steroidal Anti-Inflammatory Drug (NSAID) ketorolac was associated with significantly superior disease-free survival in the first few years after surgery. The updated analysis confirmed that the benefit appears in the 9-18 month hazards and is of magnitude 4 – 6 fold, consistent with the early report. [27] This finding is in keeping with a number of recent reports suggesting that surgery may be less successful in patients with a pre-existing elevation of some inflammatory scores, such as the neutrophil/lymphocyte ratio (NLR), the prognostic value of which was observed as well in mastectomy as in conservative breast cancer surgery. [28-29] Also, triple negative breast cancer (TNBC) patients have frequency of 12% in US population, 25% among African Americans and even more in Sub-Saharan Africa populations. [30] TNBC is looked upon by clinicians as a "bad tumour" with high recurrence rate in spite of adjuvant chemotherapy. Thais pessimistic viewpoint seems justified since in the USA, TNBC has 12% incidence but accounts for approximately 20% of mortality in breast cancer. Recurrence dynamics of TNBC patients displays a dominant early peak that looks remarkably similar to the no-ketorolac group in the study by Forget and colleagues. [26] TNBC, therefore, appears to be an ideal study group with which to test the benefit of perioperative ketorolac in a clinical trial. [31] Intraoperative NSAIDs administration has been associated with a lower incidence of early detection of postoperative distant metastases. As a consequence, it could be assumed that the effect of ketorolac may be higher in the subgroup of Nigerian patients with the highest risk of early recurrence. [32] It may be worthwhile to test the possible beneficial effect of perioperative ketorolac (a cheap and affordable NSAID) in a clinical trial among breast cancer patients of African descent. It makes an economic, public health and humanitarian sense for grant providers to fund a clinical trial on this cheap and readily available medication among patients in developing countries who may not be fortunate enough like their counterparts in the developed world to afford more expensive adjuvant and adjuvant hormone therapy.

References

1. Chalmers TC, Smith H Jr, Blackburn B, Silverman B, Schroeder B, Reitman D, Ambroz A (1981). "A method for assessing the quality of a randomized control trial". Controlled Clinical Trials 2 (1): 31–49.

2. Varughese J, Richman, S Cancer Care Inequity for Women in Resource-Poor Countries. Rev Obstet Gynecol. 2010 Summer; 3(3): 122–132.

3. Ihezue CH, Ugwu BT, Nwana EJ. Breast cancer in Highlanders. Nigerian J Surg Sci 1994; 4: 1-4.

4. Quinn M, Allen E. Changes in incidence of and mortality from breast cancer in England and Wales since introduction of screening. BMJ 1995; 311: 1391-1395.

5. Walker AR, Adam FI, Walker BF. Breast cancer in black African Women: a changing situation. J R Soc Health. 2004; 124: 81-85.

6. Gukas ID, Jennings BA, Leinster SJ, Harvey I. A theme issue by, for, and about Africa: collaborative work between Nigeria and UK on breast cancer has been successful (BMJ. 2005; 331(7519):779.

7. Okobia MN. Cancer care in sub-Saharan Africa—urgent need for population-based cancer registries. Ethiop J Health Dev 2003; 17: 89-98.

8. Osaro E, Charles AT. The challenges of meeting the blood transfusion requirements in Sub-Saharan Africa: the need for the development of alternatives to allogenic blood. J Blood Med. 2011; 2:7-21.

9. Akinbami A, Popoola A, Adediran A, Dosunmu A, Oshinaike O, Adebola P, Ajibola S. Full blood count pattern of pre-chemotherapy breast cancer patients in Lagos, Nigeria. *Caspian J Intern Med.* 2013 Winter; 4(1):574-579.

10. Adebamowo CA, Akarolo-Anthony S. Cancer in Africa: opportunities for collaborative research and training. Afr J Med Med Sci 2009; 38 (2):5-13.

11. Olken BA (2007). "Monitoring corruption: evidence from a field experiment in Indonesia". Journal of Political Economy 115 (2): 200–249

12. Bekelman JE, Li Y, Gross CP (2003). "Scope and impact of financial conflicts of interest in biomedical research: a systematic review". J Am Med Assoc 289 (4): 454–65.

13. Yitschaky O, Yitschaky M, Zadik Y (May 2011). "Case report on trial: Do you, Doctor, swear to tell the truth, the whole truth and nothing but the truth?" (PDF). J Med Case Reports 5 (1): 179.

14. Wilmshurst, P. (1997), 'Scientific imperialism. If they won't benefit from the findings, poor people in the developing world shouldn'b be used in research', British Medical Journal, 314, 840-841.

15. Mudur, G. (1997), 'India to control foreign research involving Indian patients', British Medical Journal, 314, 165.

16. Lurie, P. and Wolfe, S.M. (1997), 'Unethical trials of interventions to reduce perinatal transmission of the human immunodeficiency virus in developing countries', New England Journal of Medicine, 337, 853-856.

17. Mabey, D. (1996), 'Importance of clinical trials in developing countries', Lancet, 348, 9035,1113-4.

18. Levine, R.J. (1986), Ethics and regulation of clinical research. 2nd edition, Baltimore-Munich, Urban & Schwarzenberg.

19. Lie, R.K. (Forthcoming), 'Ethical issues in international collaborative trials', in Mordini, E. (ed.),Rome.

20. Freedman, B. (1992), 'A response to a purported ethical difficulty with randomized clinical trials involving cancer patients', Journal of Clinical Ethics, 3, 231-234.

21. Garner, P., Torres, T.T. and Alonso, P. (1994), 'Trial design in developing countries', British Medical Journal, 309, 6958, 825-6.

22. Gbolade, B.A. (1997), 'Exploitative collaborative research must be discouraged', British Medical Journal, 314, 7090, 1347.

23. Angell, M. 'The ethics of clinical research in the Third World', New England Journal of Medicine 1997; 337, 847-849.

24. Harford JB, Otero IV, Anderson BO, Cazap E, Gradishar WJ, Gralow JR, Kane GM, Niëns LM, Porter PL, Reeler AV, Rieger PT, Shockney LD, Shulman LN, Soldak T, Thomas DB, Thompson B, Winchester DP, Zelle SG, Badwe RA. Problem solving for breast health care delivery in low and middle resource countries (LMCs): consensus statement from the Breast Health Global Initiative. Breast. 2011 Apr;20 Suppl 2:S20-29.

25. Bhurgri Y, Nazir K, Shaheen Y, et al. Pathoepidemiology of cancer corpus uteri in Karachi South "1995–1997" Asian Pac J Cancer Prev. 2007;8:489–494.

26. Forget P, Vandenhende J, Berliere M, Machiels JP, Nussbaum B, Legrand C, De Kock M. Do intraoperative analgesics influence breast cancer recurrence after mastectomy? A retrospective analysis. Anesth. Analg. 2010;110:1630–1635.

27. Retsky, Michael, Romano Demicheli, William Hrushesky, Patrice Forget, Marc Kock, Isaac Gukas, Rick Rogers, Michael Baum, Vikas Sukhatme, and Jayant VaidyaReduction of breast cancer relapses with perioperative non-steroidal anti-inflammatory drugs: New findings and a review. Curr. Med. Chem. 2013;20:4163–4176.

28. Forget P, Machiels JP, Coulie PG, Berliere M, Poncelet AJ, Tombal B, Stainier A, Legrand C, Canon JL, Kremer Y, De Kock M. Neutrophil: Lymphocyte Ratio and Intraoperative Use of Ketorolac or Diclofenac are Prognostic Factors in Different Cohorts of Patients Undergoing Breast, Lung, and Kidney Cancer Surgery. Ann Surg Oncol. 2013;S650-660.

29. Demicheli R, Retsky MW, Hrushesky WJ, Baum M, Gukas ID, Jatoi I. Racial disparities in breast cancer outcome: insights into host-tumor interactions. Cancer. 2007;110:1880-1888.

30. Ikpatt OF, Ndoma-Egba R. Oestrogen and progesterone receptors in Nigerian breast cancer: relationship to tumour histopathology and survival of patients. Cent Afr J Med. 2003;49:122–126.

31. Retsky M, Rogers R, Demicheli R, Hrushesky WJ, Gukas I, Vaidya JS, Baum M, Forget P, Dekock M, Pachmann K. NSAID analgesic ketorolac used perioperatively may suppress early breast cancer relapse: particular relevance to triple negative subgroup. Breast Cancer Res Treat. 2012;134(2):881-888.

32. Forget P, De Kock M. Perspectives in anaesthesia for cancer surgery. J Cancer Res Clin Oncol. 2014 Mar;140(3):353-359.

Chapter 9

Failure in Stewardship in the Management of Breast Cancer by the Nigerian Government

Nigeria, known as "the Giant of Africa", is the most populous country in Africa and the seventh most populous country in the world with about 160 million people and more than 250 ethnic groups.[1] The rating by the United Nations Human Poverty Index in 1999 revealed that Nigeria has been ranked among the poorest nations in the world. Per capita annual income is estimated at 692 USD, with an estimated two-thirds of the population living in poverty. Although the recurrent expenditure on health has risen significantly over the years, healthcare delivered to Nigerians remains quite suboptimal.[2] The Nigerian health service is the responsibility of the Federal, State and Local Governments.[3] Over the years, the amount of budgetary allocation for health is quadrupled, yet corruption and failure in stewardship by those responsible for the health ministry has robbed Nigerians of an effective healthcare delivery system. Nigeria although oil rich has been impoverished by corrupt politicians. This has had a significant negative effect on the socioeconomic status of the average Nigerian; poor and limited access to healthcare with attendant high incidence of under diagnosis and delayed diagnosis of breast cancer among Nigeria women. Breast cancer is an established health priority in many developed countries. This has shown many dividends in reduction of the incidence and disease improvement, due to early detection which has often resulted in increase in survival among those diagnosed with breast cancer, as well as reduction in breast cancer related mortality. In Nigeria and many other developing countries, more attention is paid to communicable diseases. Our overdependence on foreign aid to run many health programs compels us to align our priorities to that of the donors. It is worthy to note that in the early 1970's when Nigeria had a responsive government, the bill of all patients treated for cancer was often forwarded to the western regional government under the leadership of Chief Obafemi Awolowo, and the hospital were often refunded within a month. Unfortunately today, despite our national budget in trillions of naira, there is not enough to pay for the health bill of citizens particularly those living with cancer. Beginning from 1960, the Nigerian government tried to curb breast cancer disease with the establishment of cancer registries in the Department of Pathology of the University College Hospital, Ibadan. This effort was directed at recording cancer incidences for use by health planners and research purposes. According to Lambo,[5] there are only 6 laboratories in Nigeria and out of the estimated 4 million Nigerians requiring radiotherapy, only 15% have access to facilities. To buttress the healthcare delivery services, a committee was set up by the Federal Ministry of Health to draw a National Cancer Policy after the World Cancer Congress in 2006, with the theme *"bridging the gap and transforming knowledge into action"*. However, up till 2007 when the Federal government inaugurated the National Commission on Cancer Control and a National policy on reproductive health and strategic framework, no item on the agenda was implemented. Analysis of data from two population based cancer registries in Nigeria; the Ibadan Population Based Cancer Registry (IBCR) and the Abuja Population Based Cancer Registry (ABCR) covering a 2 year period 2009-2010, suggested a substantial increase in incidence of breast cancer in recent times and highlights the need for high quality regional cancer registries in Nigeria and other SSA countries.[6] The national minimum wage in Nigeria currently stands at N18,000; an equivalent of $90 or £72. The cheapest and effective anti-cancer combination therapy (3 weekly cycle) costs a lot more than the national minimum wage. With a complete therapy of newer drugs costing up to 1-2 million, majority of Nigerians just cannot afford them, with a negative effect on adherence. A significant number of Nigerian women with breast cancer (80%) are likely to miss their treatment due to unaffordability. These helpless women often return to hospital in the terminal stages of their disease - a time when unfortunately little can be done to help them.[7]

The National Health Insurance Scheme (NHIS) was set up to ideally provide a comprehensive range of health services to the vast majority of

Nigerians. The scheme was set up to ensure that every Nigerian has access to good healthcare services. The law setting up the NHIS defines the role of the federal government to include coordinating the affairs of the university teaching hospitals and federal medical centers (tertiary healthcare), while the state government manages the various general and specialist hospitals (secondary healthcare), and the local government focus on dispensaries (primary healthcare). The total expenditure on healthcare as a percentage of GDP was 4.6%, while the percentage of federal government expenditure on healthcare is about 1.5%.[8] However, the NHIS has not been meeting its mandate due to limited coverage. The majority of those enrolled on the scheme are government workers and a few private establishments, with the majority of Nigerians having no access to this service.[9] Statistics from the Federal Ministry of Health shows that it contributed an insignificant 2% of the financing of health needs of the nation between 2003 and 2005. The scheme does not generally cover the disbursement of the drugs required for cancer treatment by most healthcare providers. With the rising incidence of cancers in Nigeria, the need for this facility will continue to grow. For our population, at least one radiation centre should be available in each state of the federation, while a congested place like Lagos should have several of this facility.

Nigeria has several peculiarities with regards to breast cancer; it has the highest prevalence of ailments affecting women (HIV, malaria and TB); women with breast cancer (aged 30 and more) face an increasing physical and emotional stress; high incidence of delayed presentation to clinical setting at an advanced stage (tumors are bulky and scirrhous); suboptimal health system to effectively manage the increasing cancer burden in the female population; an aggressive disease course partly due to high diagnosis among young women (more than 12% of young women are less than 30 years and premenopausal women with a peak age of 42.6 years) and the high incidence of poor prognosis associated triple negative breast cancer; poor awareness, poor diagnostic infrastructure (the detection, diagnosis and staging of breast cancer is dependent on typical investigations like biopsy, X-rays, abdominal USG scan), unavailability of cutting edge treatment (limited use of mammography, CT, flow cytometry, frozen section histology, nuclear medicine facilities); poor access to modern and advanced third generation technology and medication, poor access to hospitals particularly in rural communities; increasing incidence of male breast cancer incidence; poor treatment compliance in the few treatment centres with majority of women dying due to poor follow up; unavailability of evidence- based multimodal therapy combinations including mastectomy, chemotherapy, radiotherapy and adjuvant hormonal treatment therapy; affordability challenge and access to costly cancer drugs which is not within reach of a vast majority of patients, uneven distribution and poor access to radiation therapy, and other specialized treatments between urban and rural health facilities.

References

1. Federal Research Division. Country profile: Nigeria. USA: Federal Research Division, Library of Congress; 2008.

2. Bakare AS, Olubokun S. Health care expenditure and economic growth in Nigeria: an empirical study. J Emerg Trends Econ Manage Sci. 2011; 2(2): 83-87.

3. Rais Akhtar; Health Care Patterns and Planning in Developing Countries, Greenwood Press, 1991:264.

4. Lambo, E. O. (2007). "Press Release on State of Health in Nigeria. Retrieved on 28th Aug 2007 from google online database.

5. Jedy-Agba EE[1], Curado MP, Oga E, Samaila MO, Ezeome ER, Obiorah C, Erinomo OO, Ekanem IO, Uka C, Mayun A, Afolayan EA, Abiodun P, Olasode BJ, Omonisi A, Otu T, Osinubi P, Dakum P, Blattner W, Adebamowo CA. The role of hospital-based cancer registries in low and middle income countries-The Nigerian Case Study. Cancer Epidemiol. 2012;36(5):430-435.

6. Arowolo OA, Akinkuolie AA, Adisa AO, Obonna GC, Olasode BJ. (2012) Neglected Giant Fibroadenoma of the Breast presenting as Fungating Breast Cancer in a Premenarchal Nigerian Teenager. *West African Journal of Medicine* 31(3):211-213.

7. Ronald J. Vogel; Financing Health Care in Sub-Saharan Africa Greenwood Press, 1993: 18.

8. Gukas ID, Jennings BA, Mandong BM, et al. Clinicopathological features and molecular markers of breast cancer in Jos, Nigeria. West Afr J Med. 2005; 24:209–213.

Chapter 10

Socioeconomic Factors and Unaffordability of Breast Cancer Treatment in Nigeria.

The national minimum wage in Nigeria currently stands at N18,000; an equivalent of $90 or £72. The cheapest and most effective anti-cancer combination therapy (3weekly cycle) costs a lot more than the national minimum wage. Breast cancer treatment is expensive and above the reach of most Nigerians. According to the United Nation's Human Development Report in 2003, the bottom 25 ranked nations (151st to 175th) were all African. Poverty, illiteracy, malnutrition and inadequate water supply and sanitation, as well as poor health, affect a large proportion of the people who reside in the African continent. About 80.5% of the sub Saharan Africa population live on less than $2.50 per person per day in 2005. Africa faces several daunting challenges with regards to access to basic health services unlike their counterparts in most developed countries of the world. The healthcare system and infrastructure are suboptimal. This is often due to fundamental limitations in funding, lack of adequate qualified healthcare professional and equipment as well as deep rooted, institutionalized and chronic corruption among the political class and bureaucratic compensation and corruption among civil servants. Africa remains the world's most corrupt continent. Corruption is the abuse of entrusted power for private gain, in public and private sectors. Corruption is a cankerworm that continues to weaken societies, ruins lives, and impedes development in the African continent. This is further compounded by the high incidence of infectious diseases (HIV, TB and Malaria). Africa is plagued by poverty, malnutrition, poor sanitation, disease, high mortality rate, conflict, wars and crime. These challenges have a significant negative effect on life expectancy in the continent. Breast cancer chemotherapy in Nigeria in not cheap. A bottle of chemotherapeutic drugs like Adriamycin and Eprirubicin cost N2,000 and N10,000 respectively. Patients who requires Tamoxifen can spend up to N36,000 each year. On the average, patients are expected to use six courses of this agent every three weeks with an average total cost of N80,000 and N100,000 on drugs alone. Although a cheaper drug like cyclophosphamide exist (N400 per tablet), it is rarely prescribed. Patients that require surgery spend on the average N15,000 on lumpectomy, while mastectomy cost on the minimum about N50,000. Radiotherapy is in most cases not affordable to majority of breast cancer women. Twenty sessions can cost up to N100,000 and above. Even radiotherapy for cervical cancer costs about N50,000 and above. Cost of these services are often higher in private cancer clinics. For women who requires targeted therapy for HER 2+ breast cancer can spend N400,000 for a complete dosage of Herceptin for one month, and N4.8 million for a year treatment. Facts and figures released on 2013 World Cancer Day celebration by the Union for International Cancer Control (UICC), and the International Agency for Research on Cancer (IARC) indicates that 1.5 million lives, which would have been lost to cancer, could be saved per year if decisive measures are taken to achieve the World Health Organization's (WHO) '25 by 25' target; to reduce premature deaths due to non-communicable diseases (NCDs) by 25 per cent by 2025. Currently, 7.6 million people die from cancer worldwide every year, out of which, four million people die prematurely (aged 30 to 69 years). Socioeconomic factors have been shown to lead to late stage diagnosis and limited access to quality health (Smith-Bindman et al., 2006).

Observation from the US indicates that of women born and raised in the United States, Black women have a lower incidence rate of breast cancer but poorer survival than white women.[1] The differences in outcomes were still observed between black and white patients after accounting for stage, socioeconomic status and age.[2-3] In Nigeria, breast cancer control is often a lower priority issue creating challenges for the prevention, early diagnosis, and treatment of breast cancer. Training and education are vital components of efforts to tackle this problem.[4] Poorer survival has been observed among Black women compared with their White counterparts. A report that investigated the prognostic factors for breast cancer indicated that sociodemographic variables appeared to act largely through racial differences in stage at diagnosis, which may be amenable to change through improved access to, and use of screening for Black women.[5] Factors associated with cancer staging were differentially expressed in Blacks and Whites. Indicators of access to healthcare, a lack of mammograms, and an increased body mass index significantly contributed to stage differences in Blacks, whereas income was marginally associated with stage for whites only.[6] A number of factors have been implicated as the cause of poorer survival for Black women, including clinical and pathologic features of the disease that are indicative of poor prognosis; economic resource inequalities and differences in treatment access and efficacy.[7] SES replaces race as a predictor of worse outcome after women who are diagnosed with breast carcinoma in many studies. However, Black women present with more advanced disease that appear more aggressive biologically, and they present at a younger age compared with White women.[8-9]

Breast cancer constitutes a major public health issue globally with over 1 million new cases diagnosed annually, resulting in over 400,000 annual deaths and about 4.4 million women living with the disease. It also affects one in eight women during their lives. It is the commonest site specific malignancy affecting women and the most common cause of cancer mortality in women worldwide. It is the most common cancer in women, but it can also appear in men. The five-year survival rate for breast cancer patients in the United States exceeds 85 percent, while in Nigeria it is a dismal 10 percent. Breast cancer is responsible for about 16% of all cancer related deaths in Nigeria.[10] Breast cancer is now an epidemic, posing a serious threat to the health of women of all races globally. In Nigeria, cervical cancer was the commonest cause of cancer- related deaths among women for several decades but breast cancer is now the leading cause of cancer related deaths among Nigerian women. This is not due to a reduction in cervical cancer, but an increase in the incidence of breast cancer. Breast cancer is commonly seen in four stages that represents its progression. In stage I, the disease is confined entirely to the breast. The cancer usually start as a very tiny growth that cannot be felt but can be detected with imaging tests such as mammography and ultrasound. At this first stage, treatment is usually curative and more than 95% of those so detected will survive the disease beyond 5 years. Stage II is a cancer that has involved lymph nodes in the armpit of the same side of the breast, while stage III disease has involved the muscles under the breast. Stages II and

III therefore require very aggressive treatment using different modalities to contain the spread of the disease. It is however difficult to cure a patient in stage IV because the disease has spread to involve other organs in the body such as the lungs, liver, bones, the brain or the spine. There are many risk factors that have been associated with breast cancer; being a female, the chance of getting it increases with the age of the woman, history of breast cancer in close relatives especially in mothers and siblings, early onset of menstrual periods before the age of 12 or reaching menopause after the age of 55, prolonged period of estrogen exposure in females, overweight, using hormone replacement therapy, taking birth control pills, drinking alcohol, not having children or having your first child after age 35 or having dense breasts.

The incidence of cancers is rising worldwide. A steady increase in incidence has been observed in most developed and developing countries. Apart from incidence, cancer related deaths are also increasing. In 2008 alone, up to 7.6 million people died from cancers all over the world with about 70% of these deaths occurring in developing countries. In Nigeria, it is estimated that more than 250,000 new cases of cancers are diagnosed every year and up to 10,000 Nigerians die each year from cancer-related causes. These estimates may not be a reflection of the true picture as they are often largely based on hospital generated data without provision for the many cases that do not present in hospitals, those managed by traditional medicine practitioners, as well as the many cases of misdiagnosis in our numerous peripheral hospitals. There are over 230,000 new cases of breast cancer each year in the United States as of 2015. About 40,000 fatalities occur in the U.S. every year from this particular form of cancer.[11] The probability of getting breast cancer increases with age, and in the U.S. approximately one out of eight women will get breast cancer at some point in their lives. The physical, emotional and financial cost of this disease is staggering. The incidence of cancer continues to rise all over the world and current projections show that there will be 1.27 million new cases and almost 1 million deaths by 2030. In view of the rising incidence of cancer in sub Saharan Africa, urgent steps are needed to guide appropriate policy, health sector investment and resource allocation. Information provided by HBCR is beneficial and can be utilized for the improvement of cancer care delivery systems in low and middle income countries where there are no population based cancer registries.[12]

Metastatic disease is common in Nigeria and treatment is limited due to resource limitations. Improved awareness of the disease is advocated to reduce late presentation.[13] There is need to organize wider scale suitable methods for early detection of these diseases.[14-19] The relative frequencies of breast cancer among other female cancers, from cancer registries in Nigeria are 35.3% in Ibadan, 28.2% in Ife-Ijesha, 44.5% in Enugu, 17% in Eruwa, 37.5% in Lagos, 20.5% in Zaria and 29.8% in Calabar.[20] The predominant feature of late presentation of breast cancer had been reported over three decades in Nigeria.[10, 20-21]

References

1. Smigal C, Jemal A, Ward E, et al. Trend in breast cancer by race and ethnicity: Update 2006. Cancer J Clin. 2006; 56:168-183.

2. Newman LA, Griffith KA, Jatoi I, et al. Meta-analysis of survival in African American and white American patients with breast cancer: Ethnicity compared with socioeconomic status. J Clin Oncol. 2006; 24:1342–1349.

3. Chlebowski RT, Chen Z, Anderson GL, et al. Ethnicity and breast cancer: Factors influencing differences in incidence and outcome. J Natl Cancer Inst. 2005; 97:439–448.

4. Nwogu C, Mahoney M, George S, Dy G, Hartman H, Animashaun M, Popoola A, Michalek A. Promoting cancer control training in resource limited environments: Lagos, Nigeria. J Cancer Educ. 2014; 29(1):14-18.

5. Eley JW, Hill HA, Chen VW, et al. Racial differences in survival from breast cancer: Results of the National Cancer Institute Black/White Cancer Survival Study. JAMA. 1994; 272:947–954.

6. Hunter CP, Redmond CK, Chen VW, Austin DF, Greenberg RS, Correa P, Muss HB, Forman MR, Wesley MN, Blacklow RS, et al.Breast cancer: factors associated with stage at diagnosis in black and white women. Black/White Cancer Survival Study Group. J Natl Cancer Inst. 1993;85(14):1129-1137.

7. Dignam JJ. Differences in breast cancer prognosis among African-American and Caucasian women. CA Cancer J Clin. 2000;50(1):50-64.

8. Cross CK, Harris J, Recht A. Race, socioeconomic status, and breast carcinoma in the U.S: what have we learned from clinical studies. Cancer. 2002; 95(9):1988-1999.

9. Joslyn SA, West MM. Racial differences in breast carcinoma survival. Cancer. 2000; 88(1):114-123.

10. Adisa AO, Arowolo OA, Akinkuolie AA, Titiloye NA, Alatise OI, Lawal OO, Adesunkanmi AR. Metastatic breast cancer in a Nigerian tertiary hospital. *Afr Health Sci*. 2011; 11(2):279-284.

11. Abimbola Oluwatosin, Oladimeji Oladepo. Knowledge of breast cancer and its early detection measures among rural women in Akinyele Local Government Area, Ibadan, Nigeria. BMC Cancer 2006; 6: 271.

12. Awodele O, Adeyomoye AA, Awodele DF, Fayankinnu VB, Dolapo DC. Cancer distribution pattern in south-western Nigeria. Tanzan J Health Res. 2011 ; 13(2):125-131.

13. Adesunkanmi AR, Lawal OO, Adelusola KA, Durosimi MA. The severity, outcome and challenges of breast cancer in Nigeria. *Breast*. 2006; 15:399–409.

14. Adisa AO, Lawal OO, Adesunkanmi ARK. (2008) Paradox of wellness and nonadherence among Nigerian women on breast cancer chemotherapy. *Journal of Cancer Research and Therapeutics*. 2008; 4(3):107-110.

15. Nggada HA, Yawe KD, Abdulazeez J, Khalil MA. Breast cancer burden in Maiduguri, North Eastern Nigeria. Breast J. 2008;14(3):284-286.

16. Anyanwu SN, Egwuonwu OA, Ihekwoaba EC. Acceptance and adherence to treatment among breast cancer patients in Eastern Nigeria. Breast. 2011; 20 (2):S51-53.

17. Lawani J, Ngu VA, Osunkoya BO. A clinico-pathological review o malignant disease of the breast in the University College Hospital. Nigerian Medical journal. 1973; 3:182–187.

18. Chiedozie C. Breast Cancer in Nigeria. Cancer. 1985; 55:653–657.

Chapter 11

Challenge of Increasing Incidence of Risk Factors for Breast Cancer in Nigeria

A risk factor is anything that affects the chance of a person getting a disease. Different cancers have different associated risk factors. However, many women may have one or more breast cancer risk factors but yet never develop the disease. Also, many women with breast cancer have no apparent risk factors (other than being female and aging). Also when a woman with risk factors develops breast cancer, it is difficult to conclusively prove how the factors might have contributed. Some risk factors such as a person's gender, age and race are constant variables while others are linked to cancer predisposition factors in the environment. Also some breast cancer risk factors are associated with high risk personal behaviors, including alcohol consumption, cigarette smoking and unsafe diet.

Obesity is associated with poorer outcomes in patients with hormone receptor positive breast cancers, but this association is not well established for women with triple-negative breast cancers (TNBC). Overweight is an independent prognostic factor of OS in all women with TNBC, and menopause status may be a mitigating factor. Among premenopausal women, overweight women are at a greater risk of poor prognosis than normal weight women. If validated, these findings should be considered in developing preventive programs.[1-2] A previous case-control study that evaluated the role of anthropometric variables in breast cancer susceptibility in an indigenous sub Saharan African population drawn from Midwestern and South Eastern Nigeria among 250 women with breast cancer, and 250 age-matched women without breast cancer indicated that the waist: hip ratio is a significant predictor of breast cancer risk in Nigerian women.[3] A previous report involving 1,233 invasive breast cancer Nigerian women, and 1,101 controls indicated that the influence of height on breast cancer risk was quite strong.[4]

The role of physical activity in breast cancer prevalence has been speculated. Evidence in Africa from 2011 to 2013 involving 558 cases and 1,014 controls recruited into the African Breast Cancer Study in Nigeria, Cameroon, and Uganda in which participants completed a culturally tailored Physical Activity (PA) questionnaire that assesses habitual PA the year before diagnosis/interview. PA sub-scores (housework, occupational, and leisure PA), and a total PA score were calculated (metabolic equivalent of task, MET-hours/day). Multiple logistic regressions were performed, adjusting for age, body mass index (BMI), study sites, and menopausal status. The models were then stratified by BMI. PA of African women mainly consists of housework and work- related activities. The preliminary data show that PA may be significantly associated with reduced breast cancer risk.[5] Alcohol drinking is linked to the development of breast cancer. However, there is little knowledge about the impact of alcohol consumption on breast cancer risk among African women. A case-control study of 4,727 African women from Nigeria, Cameroon, and Uganda showed a positive relationship between breast cancer and alcohol drinking. Overall, the odds of having breast cancer were 62% higher among women who ever consumed alcohol than among non-drinkers.[6]

Parity may have different roles in the development of PABC versus other premenopausal breast cancer in Nigerian women. Prospective mothers with multiple births and a family history of breast cancer may have an elevated risk of breast cancer during their immediate postpartum period.[7]

Table 2: Risk factors for Breast Cancer

- Age (>40 years)
- Family History of Breast Cancer
- Female gender
- Race and ethnicity
- Exposure to Radiation (significant chest irradiation)
- Genetic Risk Factors (presence of breast cancer susceptibility genes; BRCA 1 (80% with range 56-84%),[8] BRCA 2 (Familial Breast Cancer, 2013), TP53 [9] and CHEK 2.[10]

- Family history of breast cancer (Having one first degree relative (mother, sister, or daughter) with breast cancer approximately doubles a woman's risk. Having 2 first degree relatives increases her risk about 3-fold).
- Prolonged (5-10 years) Hormonal Replacement Therapy (HRT) (30% increased risk with long-term use) [8]
- Oral Contraceptive (OC) use (risk is low and removed once discontinued)
- Reproductive history (> 30 years for first pregnancy)
- Treatment with Diethylstilbestrol (DES) which reduces the chance of miscarriage.
- Obesity (including post menopausal obesity particularly around waist)
- Alcohol use
- Lack of exercises
- Breastfeeding
- Breast Architecture (Women with dense breasts on mammogram have a risk of breast cancer that is 1.2 to 2 times that of women with average breast density).
- Parity (null parity) and having a first child after age 30 have a slightly higher breast cancer risk.
- Proliferative lesions with atypia such as atypical ductal hyperplasia (ADH) and atypical lobular hyperplasia (ALH). These are overgrowth of cells in the ducts or lobules of the breast tissue which increases the breast cancer risk (3.5 to 5 times higher than normal).
- Presence of proliferative lesions without atypia (Usual ductal hyperplasia (without atypia), radial scar, sclerosing adenosis, fibroadenoma and *papillomatosis*). These conditions are associated with excessive growth of cells in the ducts or lobules of the breast tissue and increase the risk of breast cancer slightly (1.5 to 2 times normal).

- Menstrual History (menarche before 12 years) and menopause after 55 years.
- Presence of benign breast conditions (Fibrosis, presence of cysts, squamous and apocrine metaplasia, mild hyperplasia, epithelial related calcifications ductal ectasia, presence of single papilloma, non-sclerosing adenosis, benign phyllodes tumor, fat necrosis, periductal fibrosis and presence of other benign tumors such as lipoma, hamartoma, hemangioma, neurofibroma and adenomyoepthelioma.

A previous case-control study that evaluated the role of anthropometric variables in breast cancer susceptibility in an indigenous sub Saharan African population drawn from Midwestern and South Eastern Nigeria among 250 women with breast cancer, and 250 age- matched women without breast cancer indicated that the Waist: Hip ratio is a significant predictor of breast cancer risk in Nigerian women.[3] A previous report involving 1,233 invasive breast cancer Nigerian women and 1,101 controls indicates that influence of height on breast cancer risk was quite strong.[4] The role of physical activity (PA) in breast cancer prevalence has been speculated. PA of African women mainly consists of housework and work-related activities. The preliminary data show that PA may be significantly associated with reduced breast cancer risk.[5] Obesity is associated with poorer outcomes in patients with hormone receptor positive breast cancers, but this association is not well established for women with triple-negative breast cancers (TNBC). Overweight is an independent prognostic factor of OS in all women with TNBC, and menopause status may be a mitigating factor. Among premenopausal women, overweight women are at a greater risk of poor prognosis than normal weight women.[1, 11] In addition, alcohol drinking among women with BMI >25 kg/m^2, clinically defined as overweight or obese, had a greater risk of developing breast cancer. Being overweight or obese has been shown to be a risk factor for postmenopausal breast cancer.[12-13]

Numerous reasons have been put forward to explain the racial difference, including drinking habits, metabolism and genetic factors. Traditionally, alcohol consumption among African women is less common compared with those in developed countries. However, as women in Africa are increasingly influenced by western cultures and are changing their lifestyle, and as the populations in African countries are becoming more affluent, more and more women may be exposed to alcohol.[14-15] Alcohol drinking is linked to the development of breast cancer. Previous study found a positive relationship between alcohol consumption and breast cancer risk among sub Saharan African women.[16] Women's drinking patterns are influenced by the cultural norms and practices of the ethnic groups to which they belong, in addition to other environmental and biological factors. In general, alcohol drinking is less common among African women than their counterparts in North America and Europe but the prevalence rates vary by country in Africa: ever drinking prevalence ranges from <1% to over 40% and current drinking prevalence ranges from none to nearly 30%. The general trend among African women is towards greater prevalence of alcohol consumption. Alcohol consumption has been considered a plausible risk factor for breast cancer. This relationship has been confirmed in some studies.[17-18] However, the majority of these studies were conducted among women in high income countries[19-20] with few in developing countries.[21-22] There are several reported correlations between alcohol consumption and female breast cancer. These studies are largely based on studies conducted in Caucasian populations.[23-24] Few studies have investigated this relationship among African women.[25] Prior studies suggests that the carcinogenic effect of alcohol consumption is strongest between menarche and the first full term pregnancy and could be implicated in both increased risk of breast cancer and benign breast disease.[26-28] Starting to drink at a young reproductive age (<30 year, particularly during 25–29 years) was associated with an increased risk of breast cancer.[29-31] The adoption of a western lifestyle and erosion of many traditional Nigerian customs that prohibited alcohol drinking has led to drastic changes in alcohol consumption patterns, including greater drinking among young Nigerian women.[32-33] WHO data show that 25.3% of the population in Africa is displaying an increase in five year trends for recorded adult per capita alcohol consumption. Surveys from Nigeria and Uganda showed a total adult (defined as 15 years or older) per capita alcohol consumption exceeded the per capita alcohol consumption in the United States (7.50–9.99).[34] There is need for this modifiable risk factor to be addressed in breast cancer prevention programs in Nigeria.[23, 25, 35]

References

1. Hao S, Liu Y, Yu KD, Chen S, Yang WT, Shao ZM. Overweight as a Prognostic Factor for Triple-Negative Breast Cancers in Chinese Women. PLoS One. 2015;10(6):e0129741.

2. Pierobon M, Frankenfeld CL. Obesity as a risk factor for triple-negative breast cancers: a systematic review and meta-analysis. Breast Cancer Res Treat. 2013; 137(1):307-314.

3. Okobia MN, Bunker CH, Zmuda JM, Osime U, Ezeome ER, Anyanwu SN, Uche EE, Ojukwu J, Kuller LH. Anthropometry and breast cancer risk in Nigerian women. Breast J. 2006;12(5):462-466.

4. Ogundiran TO, Huo D, Adenipekun A, Campbell O, Oyesegun R, Akang E, Adebamowo C, Olopade OI. Case-control study of body size and breast cancer risk in Nigerian women. Am J Epidemiol. 2010 Sep 15; 172(6):682-690.

5. Hou N, Ndom P, Jombwe J, Ogundiran T, Ademola A, Morhason-Bello I, Ojengbede O, Gakwaya A, Huo D. An epidemiologic investigation of physical activity and breast cancer risk in Africa. Cancer Epidemiol Biomarkers Prev. 2014;23(12):2748-2756.

6. Qian F, Ogundiran T, Hou N, Ndom P, Gakwaya A, Jombwe J, Morhason-Bello I, Adebamowo C, Ademola A, Ojengbede O, Olopade OI, Huo D. Alcohol consumption and breast cancer risk among women in three sub-Saharan African countries. PLoS One. 2014 Sep 8; 9(9):e106908.

7. Hou N, Ogundiran T, Ojengbede O, Morhason-Bello I, Zheng Y, Fackenthal J, Adebamowo C, Anetor I, Akinleye S, Olopade OI, Huo D. Risk factors for pregnancy-associated breast cancer: a report from the Nigerian Breast Cancer Study. Ann Epidemiol. 2013; 23(9):551-557.

8. King MC, Marks JH, Mandell JB. New York Breast Cancer Study Group. Breast and ovarian cancer risks due to inherited mutations in *BRCA1* and *BRCA2*. *Science*. 2003; 302(5645):643-646.

9. Zghair AN, Sinha DK, Kassim A, Alfaham M, Sharma AK. Differential Gene Expression of BRCA1,ERBB2 and TP53 biomarkers between Human Breast Tissue and Peripheral Blood Samples of Breast Cancer. Anticancer Agents Med Chem. 2015 Aug 24.

10. Adank MA, Jonker MA, Kluijt I, van Mil SE, Oldenburg RA, Mooi WJ, Hogervorst FB, van den Ouweland AM, Gille JJ, Schmidt MK, van der Vaart AW, Meijers-Heijboer H, Waisfisz Q. CHEK2*1100delC homozygosity is associated with a high breast cancer risk in women. J Med Genet 2011 ;48(12):860-863.

11. Pierobon M, Frankenfeld CL. Obesity as a risk factor for triple-negative breast cancers: a systematic review and meta-analysis.Breast Cancer Res Treat. 2013; 137(1):307-314.

12. Key TJ, Appleby PN, Reeves GK, Roddam A, Dorgan JF, et al. Body mass index, serum sex hormones, and breast cancer risk in postmenopausal women. J Natl Cancer Inst 2013; 95: 1218–1226.

13. Rinaldi S, Key TJ, Peeters PH, Lahmann PH, Lukanova A, et al. (2006) Anthropometric measures, endogenous sex steroids and breast cancer risk in postmenopausal women: a study within the EPIC cohort. Int J Cancer 118: 2832–2839.

14. Akarolo-Anthony SN, Ogundiran TO, Adebamowo CA. Emerging breast cancer epidemic: evidence from Africa. *Breast Cancer Res*. 2010; 12(4):S8.

15. Martinez P, Roislien J, Naidoo N, Clausen T. Alcohol abstinence and drinking among African women: data from the World Health Surveys. BMC Public Health 2011; 11: 160.

16. Qian F, Ogundiran T, Hou N, Ndom P, Gakwaya A, Jombwe J, Morhason-Bello I, Adebamowo C, Ademola A, Ojengbede O, Olopade OI, Huo D. Alcohol consumption and breast cancer risk among women in three sub-Saharan African countries. PLoS One. 2014 Sep 8; 9(9):e106908.

17. Key J, Hodgson S, Omar RZ, Jensen TK, Thompson SG, et al. Meta-analysis of studies of alcohol and breast cancer with consideration of the methodological issues. Cancer Causes Control 2006; 17: 759–770.

18. Suzuki R, Orsini N, Mignone L, Saji S, Wolk A (2008) Alcohol intake and risk of breast cancer defined by estrogen and progesterone receptor status—a meta-analysis of epidemiological studies. Int J Cancer 122: 1832–1841.

19. Baumgartner KB, Annegers JF, McPherson RS, Frankowski RF, Gilliland FD, et al. Is alcohol intake associated with breast cancer in Hispanic women? The New Mexico Women's Health Study. Ethn Dis. 2002; 12: 460–469.

20. Yoo KY, Tajima K, Miura S, Takeuchi T, Hirose K, et al. Breast cancer risk factors according to combined estrogen and progesterone receptor status: a case-control analysis. Am J Epidemiol. 1997; 146: 307–314.

21. Bao PP, Shu XO, Gao YT, Zheng Y, Cai H, et al. Association of hormone-related characteristics and breast cancer risk by estrogen receptor/progesterone receptor status in the shanghai breast cancer study. Am J Epidemiol. 2011; 174: 661–671.

22. Nichols HB, Trentham-Dietz A, Love RR, Hampton JM, Hoang Anh PT, et al. Differences in breast cancer risk factors by tumor marker subtypes among premenopausal Vietnamese and Chinese women. Cancer Epidemiol Biomarkers Prev. 2005; 14: 41–47.

23. Kwan ML, Sternfeld B, Ergas IJ, Timperi AW, Roh JM, Hong CC, Quesenberry CP, Kushi LH. Change in physical activity during active treatment in a prospective study of breast cancer survivors. Breast Cancer Res Treat. 2012 Jan;131(2):679-690.

24. Chandran U, Hirshfield KM, Bandera EV. The role of anthropometric and nutritional factors on breast cancer risk in African-American women. Public Health Nutr. 2012; 15: 738–748.

25. Adebamowo CA. Cancer incidence in Nigeria: a report from population-based cancer registries. Cancer Epidemiol. 2012; 36(5):e271-278.

26. Colditz GA, Frazier AL (1995) Models of breast cancer show that risk is set by events of early life: prevention efforts must shift focus. Cancer Epidemiol Biomarkers Prev 4: 567–571.

27. Liu Y, Colditz GA, Rosner B, Berkey CS, Collins LC, et al. Alcohol intake between menarche and first pregnancy: a prospective study of breast cancer risk. J Natl Cancer Inst 2013; 105: 1571–1578.

28. Liu Y, Tamimi RM, Berkey CS, Willett WC, Collins LC, et al. (2012) Intakes of alcohol and folate during adolescence and risk of proliferative benign breast disease. Pediatrics 129: e1192–1198.

29. Harvey EB, Schairer C, Brinton LA, Hoover RN, Fraumeni JF Jr. Alcohol consumption and breast cancer. J Natl Cancer Inst . 1987;78: 657–661.

30. Schatzkin A, Jones DY, Hoover RN, Taylor PR, Brinton LA, et al. Alcohol consumption and breast cancer in the epidemiologic follow-up study of the first National Health and Nutrition Examination Survey. N Engl J Med. 1987; 316: 1169–1173.

31. Young TB. A case-control study of breast cancer and alcohol consumption habits. Cancer. 1989; 64: 552–558.

32. Chikere EI, Mayowa MO. Prevalence and perceived health effect of alcohol use among male undergraduate students in Owerri, South-East Nigeria: a descriptive cross-sectional study. BMC Public Health. 2011; 11: 118.

33. Ramsoomar L, Morojele NK. Trends in alcohol prevalence, age of initiation and association with alcohol-related harm among South African youth: implications for policy. S Afr Med J. 2012; 102: 609–612.

34. WHO (2011) Global status report on alcohol and health. Geneva: WHO: 1–286.

35. Chandran U, Hirshfield KM, Bandera EV. The role of anthropometric and nutritional factors on breast cancer risk in African-American women. Public Health Nutr. 2012; 15: 738–748.

Chapter 12

Challenge of Poor Awareness of Breast Self Examination (BSE)

A breast self-exam is a personal check-up carried out by a woman to look for changes or problems in the breast tissue. It is advocated that for premenopausal women a monthly self-breast exam is better done 3 to 5 days after the start of monthly menstruation, while for menopausal women exam examination can be carried out on the same day every month for consistency. Previous report indicate that most women in Nigeria, though aware of BSE and its usefulness never practice it. Those who care to practice it are ignorant of how to correctly do it. There is need for a vigorous health education programme on this subject for Nigerian women. It is hoped that this will help to reduce the morbidity and mortality associated with carcinoma of the breast.[1] Clinical Breast Examination (CBE) is a convenient and very cost effective method of detecting breast lesions in the low risk population. However, both CBE and breast ultrasonography should be done in women with high risk of breast malignancy.[2] Early detection of breast cancer plays an important role in decreasing its morbidity and mortality. Level of education, smoking habits and history of breast exam by health professionals were the factors found associated with BSE practice. Training on BSE should be given to women especially during antenatal care, in order to increase the practice of BSE thus averting the severe morbidity and mortality of breast cancer in Nigeria and other developing countries.[3] Ultrasonography like mammography, can define the parenchymal breast pattern accurately. Strong correlation exists between parenchymal breast pattern and demographic, parity variables, and breast cancer risk factors.[4]

Early detection of breast cancer plays an important role in decreasing its morbidity and mortality. Breast self-examination (BSE) awareness and practices is an inexpensive way for early detection of breast cancer that may need to be fully harnessed, particularly in Nigeria and other developing countries where budgetary allocation for health is limited.[5-6] It may be necessary for the Nigeria government to face squarely the challenges of breast cancer by including training on BSE. This should be included in the curriculum for female students in Nigeria in a bid to avert the severe morbidity and mortality of breast cancer in Nigeria.[7-10] Surveys show that performing continuous BSE causes a decrease rate of 3.1% in breast cancer cases with interfacing axillary lymph.[11] Early detection of breast cancer plays an important role in decreasing its morbidity and mortality. BSE can facilitate early diagnosis allowing for early and prompt treatment and the reduction in cancer deaths.[12] Awareness, uptake and practice of BSE in Nigeria and other developing countries is low.[13-16] BSE is simple, low-priced, secure, effective, appropriate, not associated with any side effect, can be performed effectively with minimal training, can be done at home and non-health facilities and can potentially be a feasible diagnostic tool in Nigeria and other developing countries compared with mammography and clinical breast examination.[17]

Early diagnosis of breast cancer has been related to the frequency of BSE.[18] Early diagnosis and treatment can be an important strategy to reduce cancer- related deaths, particularly in Nigeria and other low and middle income countries where the diseases is diagnosed in late stages and where resources are limited.[19-20] The Nigerian government can potentially reduce significant breast cancer-related mortality by investing on training on the techniques of BSE for health extension and community health workers, and female teachers and female community leaders as a way of reaching the wider community with this far reaching opportunity to tackle the problem in Nigeria. This is likely to result in a rise in the practice of BSE which in turn can potentially avert the severe morbidity and mortality of breast cancer. [4]

Procedure for Self Breast Examination

a. View the breasts with arms down at your sides. One breast is normally a little larger than the other, but do they appear about the same size and shape? Is the outline of each breast rounded and smooth, or are there any creases or dimples?

b. Look at your breasts for the same signs as in (a), but this time with your arms raised and your hands holding each other behind your head.

c. Repeat the visual inspection with your hands on your hips.

d. Raise your right hand above your head; with all four fingertips of your left hand, gently press the whole of your right breast, moving your fingers to the next area and using small circular movements. Feel for any lumps or thickened tissue. Repeat with the left breast and right hand.

e. Hold your right nipple between the thumb and first finger of your left hand; gently roll the nipple, feeling for any lumps or tenderness. Repeat with the left breast.

f. Lie down and stretch your left arm upwards and behind your head. Use small circular pressures with the fingertips of your right hand to examine the whole breast. Repeat with the right breast and left hand.

Table 3: Observation during Breast Self Examination (BSE) that should trigger the need for Clinical Breast Examination (CBE)

Observation during BSE	Possible Presentation requiring a CBE
Lump	• Observation of any lump (painless or painful) or hard knot found in the breast or armpit. • Any new lump or thickening that does not shrink or lessen after your next period

Change in breast Color, Size or Texture	• Observation of any change in breast size, shape or symmetry • Observation of any thickening or swelling of the breast
Changes in nipple architecture	• Redness or scaliness of the nipple or breast skin • Unusual nipple tenderness or pain • Unusual nipple retraction, drawing inward or nipple pointing to an unusual new direction
Dimpling of the skin in the breast and nipple area	• Observation of any unusual dimpling, puckering or indention in the breast • Observation of any unusual skin dimpling, skin irritation, ulceration or other change in the breast skin or nipple
Nipple discharges	• Any unusual discharges from the nipples (except for breast milk) that occur freely without any pressure or squeezing of the nipple that is dark, bloody or clear and sticky.
Lymph node changes	• Lymphoedema, axillary, infra/supraclavicular lymphadenopathy

References

1. Jebbin NJ, Adotey JM. Attitudes to, knowledge and practice of breast self-examination (BSE) in Port Harcourt. Niger J Med. 2004; 13(2):166-170.

2. Ezeonu PO, Ajah LO, Onoh RC, Lawani LO, Enemuo VC, Agwu UM. Evaluation of clinical breast examination and breast ultrasonography among pregnant women in Abakaliki, Nigeria. Onco Targets Ther. 2015 May 13;8:1025-9.

3. Obajimi MO, Adeniji-Sofoluwe AT[1], Adedokun BO, Soyemi TO, Bassey OS. Sonographic breast pattern in women in Ibadan, Nigeria. Ann Afr Med. 2014;13(4):145-150.

4. Amoran OE, Toyobo OO. Predictors of breast self-examination as cancer prevention practice among women of reproductive age-group in a rural town in Nigeria. Niger Med J. 2015;56(3):185-189.

5. Banaian SH, Kazemian A, Soleiman KH. Knowledge, attitude, practice among women referred to health centers in Broojen about screening methods of breast cancer. J Shahrekord Univ Med Sci. 2005;7:28–34.

6. Harris DM, Miller JE, Davis DM. Racial differences in breast cancer screening, knowledge and compliance. J Natl Med Assoc. 2003;95:693–701.

7. Brower V. Developing nations face challenges as breast cancer rises. J Natl Cancer Inst. 2011 Dec 21;103(24):1812-4..

8. Anim JT. Breast cancer in sub-Saharan African women. Afr J Med Med Sci. 1993 Mar;22(1):5-10.

9. González-Robledo LM, González-Robledo MC, Nigenda G, López-Carrillo L. Government actions for the early detection of breast cancer in Latin America. Future challenges. Salud Publica Mex. 2010 Nov-Dec;52(6):533-543.

10. Schwartsmann G. Breast cancer in South America: challenges to improve early detection and medical management of a public health problem. J Clin Oncol. 2001 Sep 15;19(18 Suppl):118S-124S.

11. Carelli I, Pompei LM, Mattos CS, Ferreira HG, Pescuma R, Fernandes CE, et al. Knowledge, attitude and practice of breast self-examination in a female population of metropolitan São Paulo. Breast. 2008;17:270–4.

12. Danesh A, Amiri M, Ramezani A, Tazhibi M, Ganji F. Knowledge, attitude, practice among female workers in shahrekord education

organization about breast self examination. J Shahrekord Univ Med Sci. 2002;4:47–52.

13. Agboola AO, Deji-Agboola AM, Oritogun KS, Musa AA, Oyebadejo TY, Ayoade BA. Knowledge, attitude and practice of breast self examination in female health workers in Olabisi Onabanjo University teaching hospital, Sagamu, Nigeria. Int Med J. 2007;8:5–10.

14. Akhigbe AO, Omuemu VO. Knowledge, attitudes and practice of breast cancer screening among female health workers in a Nigerian urban city. BMC Cancer. 2009;9:203.

15. Alkhasawneh LM, Akhu-Zaheya LM, Suleiman SM. Knowledge and practice of breast self-examination. J Adv Nurs. 2009;65:412–6.

16. Ibrahim NA, Odusanya OO. Knowledge of risk factors, beliefs and practices of female healthcare professionals towards breast cancer in a tertiary institution in Lagos, Nigeria. BMC Cancer. 2009;9:76.

17. Nakhichevan NO, Secginli S. Health belief related to breast self-examination in a sample of Turkish women. Oncol Nurs Forum. 2007;34:425–432.

18. Chong PN, Krishnan M, Hong CY, Swash TS. Knowledge and practice of breast cancer screening amongst public health nurses in Singapore. Singapore Med J. 2002;43:509–16.

19. Loescher L. Nursing roles in cancer prevention position statements. Semin Oncol Nurs. 2004;20:111–20.

20. Abdel-Fattah M, Zaki A, Bassili A, El-Shazly M, Tognoni G. Breast self-examination practice and its impact on breast cancer diagnosis in Alexandria, Egypt. East Mediterr Health J. 2000;6:34–40

Chapter 13

Role of Spirituality in the Delay in Seeking Care among Breast Cancer Patients

Nigeria is a highly religious nation. It is divided into a Christian dominated South and a Muslim dominated North. Religion involves a specific set of beliefs and practices, usually within an organized group. Spiritual or religious beliefs and practices can have a significant effect on patients with breast cancer (when and whether to seek medical care and in coping with their disease (spiritual coping).

Spiritual or religious beliefs and practices can have a positive effect on mental attitude; improve well-being and quality of life of women with breast cancer. Religion and spirituality plays a prominent role in the social and cultural life of Africans. Most women in Nigeria and other settings in SSA identify with a variety of faith- based groups where their leaders have a considerable measure of influence, built on a combination of trust and culture. Religious leaders in Nigeria and other settings in Africa can be empowered to provide potential access for health promotion, health education and improvement in utilization of health services. A previous report has shown that an active role in religion, reporting a lengthy duration of worship at the same place was beneficial. [1] Church, mosques and faith leaders could play a greater role in raising awareness on the potential benefits of early breast self examination, early detection, the need to continue to go for regular medical care and attention even when they believe they have been healed spiritually, and the need to seek medical attention early following breast cancer diagnosis. Religious leaders in Nigeria can potentially reach a significant number of people within a short space of time. This education and awareness is what is desperately needed in Nigeria and other settings in Africa. It can in the long term lead to increased awareness and practice of BSE among Africans women. There is a strong impact of religion on people of African descent. Faith organisations may provide potential access for health promotion and interventions related to breast cancer. [2]

In a study involving 2,154 Nigerian breast cancer patients of all ages and socio-economic groups, 87% presented in Stages III or IV, and only 13% in Stages I or II. All were questioned on their reasons for not attending hospital sooner. The most common reason for delay (963 patients, 44.7%) was fear of mastectomy. Other reasons given include preference for prayer houses or spiritual healing homes (291 patients, 13.5%), a belief that the lesion was inflammatory (183 patients, 8.5%), preference for native doctors or herbalists (497 patients, 23.1%), and economic reasons (220 patients, 10.2%). [3] Spirituality and religiosity are significant factors responsible for delay in screening for breast cancer among African American women. [4] The overall survival rate among breast cancer patient is low and patients with early breast cancer had better survival than those with advanced disease. [5] Similarly, all female breast cancer patients referred to one of the general surgery out-patient clinics of Lagos State University Teaching Hospital were interviewed to evaluate the effects of selected socio-demographic factors on late presentation and reasons why breast cancer patients delay reporting for treatment. Ignorance of the nature of illness, belief in spiritual healing, fear of mastectomy and belief in herbal treatment were the leading reasons for delay. [6] Other variables related to delays included factors such as advancing age, low socioeconomic status, fear of diagnosis, consequences of cancer treatments, shame and embarrassment, misconceptions about the aetiology of breast cancer, family priorities, denial, and spirituality including faith-influenced delays. [4] Nigeria is a highly religious and culturally sensitive nation. There is increasing advocacy for implementation of appropriate, evidence-based nursing care which include spiritually-based interventions that acknowledge the significance of God. [7,8] Nigerian women in particular and Africa in general face significant physical, emotional and social changes and difficulties following primary breast cancer diagnosis. Culturally sensitive therapeutic groups and interventions should be established to help Nigerian women with breast cancer and their spouses and families understand and cope with the disease and its long- term health and quality of life implications. [4, 9-11] Experience from Thailand indicates that patient and system delay in breast cancer care are important weaknesses of disease control. System delay in hospitals outside the university needs to be improved by a good referral system. [12]

Financial barriers limit the ability of women, especially the poorest SES group, to utilize screening and treatment services for early diagnosis and treatment of breast cancer. Interventions that will improve financial risk protection for women with breast cancer or at risk of breast cancer are needed to ensure equitable access to screening and treatment services. [13-14] Evidence from Kaduna, Nigeria on the reason for delayed treatment among symptomatic breast cancer is related to the quality of medical care, local beliefs, ignorance of the disease, and lack of acceptance of orthodox treatment. [15] It is becoming increasingly clear that for breast cancer prevention programs in Nigeria to succeed, there must in addition to breast cancer awareness and screening programs, be need to address the role of spiritual leaders and institution as well as institutional bottlenecks, the dearth of knowledge among primary care physicians and improvement in referrals from alternative practitioners and prayer houses. [16]

References

1. Allain JP, Anokwa M, Casbard A, Owusu-Ofori S, Dennis-Antwi J. (2004). Sociology and behaviour of West African blood donors: the impact of religion on human immunodeficiency virus infection. *Vox Sang*; 87(4):233-240.

2. Toni-Uebari T.K., Inusa B.P.D. (2009). The role of religious leaders and faith organisations in haemoglobinopathies: a review. *BMC Blood Disorders;* 9:6.

3. Ajekigbe AT. Fear of mastectomy: The most common factor responsible for late presentation of carcinoma of the breast in Nigeria. *Clinical Oncology*; 1991; 3(2): 78–80.

4. Gullatte MM, Phillips JM, Gibson LM. Factors associated with delays in screening of self-detected breast changes in African-American women. J Natl Black Nurses Assoc. 2006; 17(1):45-50.

5. Kene TS, Odigie VI, Yusufu LM, Yusuf BO, Shehu SM, Kase JT. Pattern of presentation and survival of breast cancer in a teaching hospital in north Western Nigeria. Oman Med J. 2010; 25(2):104-107.

6. Ibrahim NA, Oludara MA. Socio-demographic factors and reasons associated with delay in breast cancer presentation: a study in Nigerian women. Breast. 2012; 21(3):416-418.

7. Gibson LM, Hendricks CS. Integrative review of spirituality in African American breast cancer survivors. ABNF J. 2006 Spring; 17(2):67-72.

8. Polzer Casarez RL, Miles MS. Spirituality: a cultural strength for African American mothers with HIV. Clin Nurs Res. 2008 May;17(2):118-132.

9. Adisa AO, Gukas ID, Lawal OO, Adesunkanmi AR. Breast cancer in Nigeria: is non-adherence to chemotherapy schedules a major factor in the reported poor treatment outcome? *Breast J.* 2010 Mar-Apr;16(2):206-207,

10. Gullatte MM, Brawley O, Kinney A, Powe B, Mooney K. Religiosity, spirituality, and cancer fatalism beliefs on delay in breast cancer diagnosis in African American women. J Relig Health. 2010; 49(1):62-72.

11. Odigie VI, Tanaka R, Yusufu LM, Gomna A, Odigie EC, Dawotola DA, Margaritoni M. Psychosocial effects of mastectomy on married African women in Northwestern Nigeria. Psychooncology. 2010;19(8):893-897.

12. Thongsuksai P, Chongsuvivatwong V, Sriplung H. Delay in breast cancer care: a study in Thai women. Med Care. 2000; 38(1):108-114.

13. Ali R, Mathew A, Rajan B. Effects of socio-economic and demographic factors in delayed reporting and late-stage presentation among patients with breast cancer in a major cancer hospital in South India. *Asian Pac J Cancer Prev.* 2008; 9(4):703-707.

14. Okoronkwo IL, Ejike-Okoye P, Chinweuba AU, Nwaneri AC. Financial barriers to utilization of screening and treatment services

for breast cancer: an equity analysis in Nigeria. Niger J Clin Pract. 2015 Mar-Apr;18(2):287-91.

15. Ukwenya AY, Yusufu LM, Nmadu PT, Garba ES, Ahmed A. Delayed treatment of symptomatic breast cancer: the experience from Kaduna, Nigeria. S Afr J Surg. 2008; 46(4):106-110.

16. Ezeome ER. Delays in presentation and treatment of breast cancer in Enugu, Nigeria. Niger J Clin Pract. 2010; 13(3):311-316.

Chapter 14

Challenge of Increasing Incidence of Breast Cancer among Men

Male breast cancer (MBC) is an uncommon disease accounting for approximately 1% of all breast cancers diagnosed in the United States each year.[1-2] Of the 209,060 total cases of breast cancer expected in the United States in 2010, 1,970 (0.94%) will occur in men and 390 men are expected to die from the disease.[3] In contrast to western countries, the incidence of MBC in sub Saharan Africa ranges from 1.3–15%.[4-5] Male breast malignancies are rare. Cancer of the male breast accounts for about of all breast cancers.[6] A retrospective study of all cases of male breast cancer (MBC) managed in Jos University Teaching Hospital over a 17 year period (January 1987-December 2003.) indicated that out of a total of 302 cases of breast malignancies managed over the study period, twenty-six (8.6%) of these were males giving a male: female ratio of 1:10.6. All the patients had history of breast lumps, 21 (80.8%) of which were painless. Skin ulceration and axillary node enlargement were present in 19(73.1%) and 24(92.3%) respectively. Five (19.2%) were stage II; 15(57.7%) stage III and 6(23.1%) were stage IV. There were 23 (88.5%) carcinomas, 2 (7.7%) fibrosarcomas and a case of Hodgkin's lymphoma. Invasive ductal carcinoma was the most common histological type in 20 (76.9%) of all breast malignancy and 20 (87.0%) of all breast carcinomas.[4] Similarly a review of all cases of MBC seen at LAUTECH Teaching Hospital Osogbo between January 2004 and December 2006 indicated that seven (8.86%) out of seventy-nine cases of breast cancers seen are males. Ages ranged between 38 and 80 years (mean 60.5, median 65 years). They all presented with advanced lesions after a 6-36 months delay (mean-11.57 months).[7] A 20 year (1987-2006) retrospective study of all patients with breast cancer indicated that sixteen cases (18.4%) of male breast cancer were encountered. Stage IV disease was most commonly encountered (43.8%). Eleven (68.8%) patients had modified radical mastectomy.[8] Sixteen (9%) Nigerian men presented with advanced breast cancer to Ahmadu Bello University Hospital in Zaria, Nigeria over the 15 year period of 1975 to 1989. The median age was 55 years, and 14 (87.5%) of the patients had Stage IV cancer at presentation.[9] The evaluation, treatment and outcome of male patients seen with breast cancer in Zaria from 2001 to 2010 indicated that 57 male (9%) patients had breast cancer. The mean age was 59 ± 2.3 years and fifty-three (93%) patients presented with advanced disease including 15 with distant metastasis.[10] A previous report on 635 patients with histological diagnosis of breast carcinoma managed in Zaria, 57 (9.0%) were males.[10] There were 57 male patients with breast cancer which accounted for 9% of all breast cancers seen during the study period. Their mean age was 59 ± 2.3 years. The mean tumour diameter was 13 ± 2.5 cm. Fifty-three (93%) patients presented with advanced disease including 15 with distant metastasis. Four patients with stage II disease were treated with modified radical mastectomy, chemotherapy and Tamoxifen. Of the 30 patients with sage III disease that had modified radical mastectomy, complete axillary clearance and tumour free margins were achieved in 25. Overall, 21 (36.8%) patients were tumour free at one year. Overall 5 year survival was 22.8%.[11]

Male breast cancer is fast becoming a common occurrence in Nigeria. Sixteen Nigerian men presented with advanced breast cancer to Ahmadu Bello University Hospital in Zaria, Nigeria over the 15 year period 1975 to 1989; comprising 9% of patients with breast cancer seen during this period.[9] A review of all cases of MBC seen at LAUTECH Teaching Hospital Osogbo between January 2004 and December 2006 indicated that seven (8.86%) out of seventy-nine cases of breast cancers seen were males.[7] In addition, it is estimated that approximately 10% of men with breast cancer have a genetic predisposition of which BRCA2 is the most clearly associated gene mutation.[12] Associations have also been suggested with BRCA 1, P53, and CHEK 2 mutations.[13-14] A recent study revealed that having a history of breast cancer in a brother is associated with a higher risk of breast cancer than having an affected sister, suggesting that MBC has a higher genetic basis than FBC.[14] The Klinefelter syndrome, characterized by a 47-XXY karyotype, small testes, azospermia, and gynecomastia, has also been described as occurring in 3–7.5% of men with breast cancer.[13] Gynecomastia present in 6–38% of MBC patients has been described as a risk factor, although it is unclear whether gynecomastia is a risk factor for MBC or the risk factors for MBC are the same as those for gynecomastia.[14] The contributions of several other variables including smoking, alcohol consumption, and exposure to electromagnetic radiation remain uncertain.[15-16]

In sub Saharan Africa patients with MBC present late with advanced disease and associated comorbidity.[9] These patients often seek non-orthodox treatment because of poor awareness, sociocultural or religious reasons. In addition, whilst surgical therapy is readily available, other resources for breast cancer treatment may be lacking or very limited. These factors may be responsible for the poor treatment outcome among the patients.[4] The rarity of MBC results in paucity of prospective randomized studies validating the efficacy of various treatment strategies for MBC.

Nigerian male patients with breast cancer like their female counterparts present with advanced disease which is associated with poor outcome of treatment.[10] The prevalence of male breast cancer in Nigeria varies from 1.2% in Enugu[4] to 2.4% in Ibadan,[17] 3.7% in North Eastern Nigeria,[18] 3.75% in Ibadan,[19] 8.6% in Jos [4] and 9.0% in Zaira.[9] A previous study that evaluated management and outcomes among 57 male patients with breast cancer indicated a mean age was 59 ± 2.3 years and mean tumour diameter was 13 ± 2.5 cm. Fifty-three (93%) patients presented with advanced disease, including 15 with distant metastasis. Four patients with stage II disease were treated with modified radical mastectomy, chemotherapy and Tamoxifen. Of the 30 patients with sage III disease that had modified radical mastectomy, complete axillary clearance and tumor free margins were achieved in 25. Overall 21 (36.8%) patients were tumour free at one year. Overall 5 year survival was 22.8%. Male patients with breast cancer present with advanced disease which is associated with poor outcome of treatment.[12]

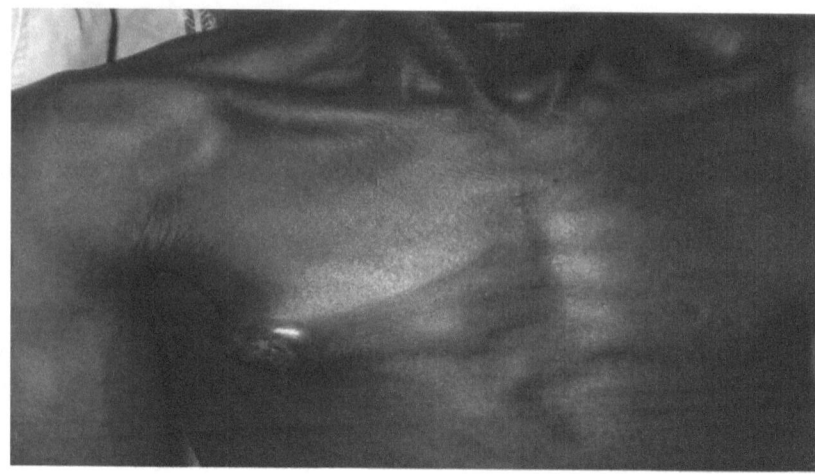

Figure 11: **A 60 year old Nigerian man with locally advanced right breast carcinoma** (Courtesy of Dr. Adewale Adisa Consultant Surgeon Department Of Surgery, Obafemi Awolowo University Ile-Ife, Nigeria)

Table 4: **Prevalence of male breast cancer in different parts of Nigeria**

Location	% Prevalence	Authors
Ibadan	3.75%	Ihekwaba, 1994 [19]
Zaria	9%	Hassan, 1995 [9]
North East Nigeria	3.7%	Dogo 2000 [18]
Jos	8.6%	Kidmas 2005 [4]
Enugu	1.2%	Ezeome 2010 [16]
Ibadan	2.4%	Ogundiran 2008 [17]

In the UK, current estimates indicate around 300 cases annually.[20] In a report from Zambia, 15% of breast cancer cases were male.[21] Previous report indicate a MBC prevalence of 9% reported from Zaria,[9] 8.6% from Jos[4] and 8% from Eastern Nigeria.[4] Similarly, prevalence of 1.47% was observed in Nnewi[22] and 2.5% in Benin.[8]

In sub Saharan Africa, patients with MBC present late with advanced disease and associated comorbidity.[4, 9, 21, 23] Evidence from previous report from Enugu[9] and Zaira[6] indicates that a significant number of MBC cases present in stage III and stage IV. Other studies from Africa reported stage IV disease in 43.8%–67.1% of their patients.[7,8,24] These patients often seek non-orthodox treatment because of poor awareness, unaffordability, socio-cultural or religious reasons. In addition, surgical therapy is not readily available particularly in rural areas coupled with the fact that other resources for breast cancer treatment may be lacking or very limited. These often result in poor outcome of treatment.[4, 9] In this series, the 5 year survival rate was 50% for stage II disease and 20.8% for advanced disease. Other studies from Nigeria indicate overall survival ranging from 6 months to 3 years.[5, 6, 7] In the study from LAUTECH, 57% of patients died from one week to seven months after diagnosis while an overall 3 year survival of 27.2% was reported from Enugu.[5] The five year OS in the patients was 22.8%. Similar poor survival rates were reported from other studies in low income countries.[9, 21, 24] In high income countries the five year OS rates for all stages of breast cancer in men range from 36%–66%, and 10 year survival rates range from 17%–52%.[25-28] Incidence rates in Egypt were 12 times that of the United States but the current incidence rate (1.42%) is only slightly higher than the U.S. rate.[29]

References

1. Nahleh ZA, Srikantiah R, Safa M, Jazieh AR, Muhleman A, Komrokji R. Male breast cancer in the Veterans Affairs population: a comparative analysis. *Cancer.* 2007; 109(8):1471–1477.

2. Contractor KB, Kaur K, Rodrigues GS, Kulkarni DM, Singhal H. "Male breast cancer: is the scenario changing. World Journal of Surgical Oncology 2008; 6: 58.

3. Jemal J, Siegel R, Xu J, Ward E. Cancer Statistics 2010. CA Cancer Journal for Clinicians 2010; 60 (5): 277–300.

4. Kidmas AT, Ugwu BT, Manasseh AN, Iya D, Opaluwa AS. Male breast malignancy in Jos University Teaching Hospital. *West African Journal of Medicine.* 2005; 24(1):36-40.

5. Ezeome ER, Emegoakor CD, Chianakwana GU, Anyanwu SNC. The pattern of male breast cancer in Eastern Nigeria: a 12 year review. *Nigerian Medical Journal.* 2010; 51:26–29.

6. Ihekwaba FN. The management of male breast cancer in Nigerians. *Postgraduate Medical Journal.* 1993; 69(813):562–565.

7. Oguntola AS, Aderonmu AO, Adeoti ML, Olatoke SA, Akanbi O, Agodirin SO. Male breast cancer in LAUTECH teaching hospital Osogbo, South Western Nigeria. *The Nigerian Postgraduate Medical Journal.* 2009; 16(2):166–170.

8. Olu-Eddo AN, Momoh MI. Clinicopathological study of male breast cancer in Nigerians and a review of the literature. *Nigerian Quarterly Journal of Hospital Medicine.* 2010; 20(3):121–124.

9. Hassan I, Mabogunje O. Cancer of the male breast in Zaria, Nigeria. *East African Medical Journal.* 1995; 72(7):457–458.

10. Ahmed A, Ukwenya Y, Abdullahi A, Muhammad I. Management and outcomes of male breast cancer in Zaria, Nigeria. *Int J Breast Cancer.* 2012; 2012:845143.

11. Adamu Ahmed, Yahaya Ukwenya, Adamu Abdullahi, Iliyasu Muhammad. (2012). Management and Outcomes of Male Breast Cancer in Zaria, Nigeria. Int J Breast Cancer; 2012: 845143.

12. Brinton LA, Carreon JD, Gierach GL, McGlynn KA, Gridley G. Etiologic factors for male breast cancer in the U.S. Veterans Affairs medical care system database. *Breast Cancer Research and Treatment.* 2010; 119(1):185–192.

13. Bevier M, Sundquist K, Hemminki K. Risk of breast cancers in families of multiple affected women and men. *Breast Cancer Research and Treatment.* 2012; 132:723–728.

14. Korde LA, Zujewski JA, Kamin L, et al. Multidisciplinary meeting on male breast cancer: summary and research recommendations. *Journal of Clinical Oncology.* 2010; 28(12):2114–2122.

15. Atalay, M. Kanlioz, and M. Altinok, "Prognostic factors affecting survival in male breast cancer," Journal of Experimental and Clinical Cancer Research. 2003; 22 (1): 29–33.

16. Ferlay J, Cancer IAFRO. GLOBOCAN 2000: cancer incidence, mortality and prevalence worldwide. IARC press; 2001.

17. Ogundiran TO, Ayandipo OO, Ademola AF, Adebamowo CA. Mastectomy for management of breast cancer in Ibadan, Nigeria. BMC Surg. 2013; 13:59.

18. Dogo D, Pindiga PU, Yawe T. Pattern of breast lesions in north eastern Nigeria. Tropical J Med Research 2000;3:14-17.

19. Ihekwaba FN. Breast cancer in men in black Africa: a report of 73 cases. J R Coll Surg Edinb. 1994; 39(6):344-347.

20. Speirs V, Shaaban AM. The rising incidence of male breast cancer. *Breast Cancer Research and Treatment*. 2009; 115(2):429–430.

21. Bhagwandin S. Carcinoma of the male breast in Zambia. *East African Medical Journal*. 1972; 49:l76–199.

22. Smigal C, Jemal A, Ward E, et al. Trend in breast cancer by race and ethnicity: Update 2006. Cancer J Clin. 2006; 56:168-183.

23. Amir H, Hirji KF. Carcinoma of the male breast in Tanzania. *Journal of the National Medical Association*. 1992; 84(4):337–340.

24. Rachid S, Yacouba H, Hassane N. Male breast cancer: 22 case reports at the National Hospital of Niamey, Niger. *The Pan African Medical Journal*. 2009; 3:15–18.

25. Fogh S, Hirsch AE, Langmead JP, et al. Use of tamoxifen with postsurgical irradiation may improve survival in estrogen and progesterone receptor-positive male breast cancer. *Clinical Breast Cancer*. 2011; 11(1):39–45.

26. Liukkonen S, Saarto T, Mäenpää H, Sjöström-Mattson J. Male breast cancer: a survey at the Helsinki University Central Hospital during 1981–2006. *Acta Oncologica*. 2010; 49(3):322–327.

27. Mauriac L, Luporsi E, Cutuli B, et al. Summary version of standard options and recommendations for non-metastatic breast cancer. *British Journal of Cancer.* 2003; 89(1):517–531.

28. Visram H, Kanji F, Dent SF. Endocrine therapy for male breast cancer: rates of toxicity and adherence. *Current Oncology.* 2010; 17(5):17–21.

29. Rennert G. Breast cancer. In: Freedman LS, Edwards BK, Ries LAG, Young JL, editors. *Cancer Incidence in Four Member Countries (Cyprus, Egypt, Israel, and Jordan) of the Middle East Cancer Consortium (MECC) Compared With US SEER.* NIH Publication; 2006: 73–79.

Chapter 15

Poor knowledge and awareness- related challenges associated with Breast Cancer

Another major challenge with breast cancer in Nigeria is the increasing detection of advanced disease in young women. Large percentage of our women presents with breast cancers in either stages III or IV. In Ile-Ife for instance, 52% of women presenting with breast cancer between 1991 and 2005 had stage IV diseases.[1] In most Western countries, breast cancer is more frequently diagnosed in older women with the peak age being in the sixth and seventh decades of life. The disease however occurs at least a decade earlier among Nigerian women. The majority of reports from Nigerian hospitals confirm the late 40s as the mean age at initial diagnosis. It is also not uncommon to find many women younger than 40 with the disease in our setting.

The poor awareness of breast cancer symptoms also contribute to this late presentation. In most instances, breast cancers starts as a painless lump. A number of Nigeria women who detect such lumps in their breasts however disregard it because it is not painful, and many will seek treatment only when the lump has grown so big to cause discomfort.[2]

A previous report to assess the knowledge of breast cancer and its early detection measures among rural women in two randomly selected health districts in Akinyele Local Government in Ibadan, Nigeria indicated that respondents lacked knowledge of vital issues about breast cancer and early detection measures.

A study was conducted in Ibadan in 2005, the investigators set out to assess the level of knowledge of breast cancer among women in the community; 65% of the women were adjudged to have poor knowledge of the symptoms that may indicate cancer of the breast. The majority who noticed a lump in their breasts delay for up to 3-6months before seeking medical attention "because it is not painful". Sadly, breast cancer usually starts as a painless lump and pain usually occurs when the disease is advanced or when infection is associated. Nigerian women should therefore learn not to disregard a painless breast lump. The fact is, a lump in the breast that starts out being very painful may not be a cancer but will equally require further examination and tests. Several reports from low and middle income countries similar to Nigeria have indicated that women who practice regular Self Breast Examination (SBE) can detect lumps at relatively early stages and seek intervention, thereby reducing the disabilities and deaths commonly associated with late presentations of the disease. Sadly, the practice of SBE is very low among Nigerian women. Some studies have reported that only 35-50% of our women, including professionals know of the benefits of SBE and only a smaller percentage practice SBE. There is therefore need to educate the populace on the benefits of this simple practice on the health of women in the Nigerian nation and other African settings. Women in the reproductive age and beyond are equally encouraged to present to a healthcare provider for a clinical breast examination since a trained personnel may be able to detect lumps in the breast or point out suspicious areas that may require further investigations. African woman aged 40 years and above should endeavour to have a check-up at least twice a year. Community dwelling women in Nigeria have poor knowledge of breast cancer, and minority practice BSE and CBE.[3] Knowledge of aetiological causes of breast cancer, including risk factors is abysmally low among Nigerian women.[4]

Report from a previous study indicates that a substantial number of Nigerian women are still ignorant of breast cancer issues.[5] There are several awareness related challenges in Nigeria. The training of healthcare workers in Nigeria needs to be optimized. Nigerian women lacked knowledge of vital issues about breast cancer and early detection measures, and health workers do not seem to have answers to the questions that breast cancer patients have.[6] Interventional studies are required to enhance the awareness of breast cancer and its early detection measures among the rural population to influence early detection of breast cancer and subsequently reduce morbidity and mortality.[7] BSE practices were found to be inadequate among secondary school and undergraduate female students in Nigeria and there is increasing advocacy to increase knowledge related to breast cancer, as well as the practice of breast self-examination.[8-9] The poor level of awareness and practice of breast screening is responsible for the late presentation of breast cancer in Nigeria.[10] Several postulations has been put forward to facilitate early detection of breast cancer in Nigeria. Public health education using the media could significantly reduce the knowledge-practice gap, and early detection of breast lump.[6,11] There is the urgent need for interventions promoting awareness of this screening procedure to the illiterate and older women.[12] Breast cancer prevention and screening are limited among African American women. Barriers include limited knowledge, lack of insurance, spiritual beliefs, and secrecy. Suggestions for promoting breast health in the Nigerian community include using culturally relevant materials and involving African men. There is need for additional research in developing a culturally- tailored breast cancer intervention.[13] Also, awareness of prophylactic mastectomy is low among patients. Education about breast cancer and methods of prevention need to be improved.[14]

References

1. Adisa AO, Lawal OO, Adesunkanmi ARK. (2008) Paradox of wellness and nonadherence among Nigerian women on breast cancer chemotherapy. *Journal of Cancer Research and Therapeutics.* 2008; 4(3):107-110.

2. Abimbola Oluwatosin, Oladimeji Oladepo. Knowledge of breast cancer and its early detection measures among rural women in Akinyele Local Government Area, Ibadan, Nigeria. BMC Cancer 2006; 6: 271.

3. Okobia M.N, Bunker C.H, Okonofua FE, Osime U. Knowledge, attitude and practice of Nigerian women towards breast cancer: A cross-sectional study. *World Journal of Surgical Oncology* 2006; 4: 11–15.

4. Aderounmu AO, Egbewale BE, Ojofeitimi EO, Fadiora SO, Oguntola AS, Asekun-Olarinmoye EO, Adeoti ML, Akanbi O. Knowledge, attitudes and practices of the educated and non-educated women

to cancer of the breast in semi-urban and rural areas of SouthWest, Nigeria. *Niger Postgrad Med J.* 2006; 13(3):182-188.

5. Azubuike S, Okwuokei S. Knowledge, attitude and practices of women towards breast cancer in Benin City, Nigeria. Ann Med Health Sci Res. 2013 3(2):155-160.

6. Bello TO, Olugbenga-Bello AI, Oguntola AS, Adeoti ML, Ojemakinde OM. Bello TO, Olugbenga-Bello AI, Oguntola AS, Adeoti ML, Ojemakinde OM. Knowledge and practice of breast cancer screening among female nurses and lay women in Osogbo, Nigeria. Niger Postgrad Med J. 2012; 19(1):19-24.

7. Oluwatosin OA, Oladepo O. Knowledge of breast cancer and its early detection measures among rural women in Akinyele Local Government Area, Ibadan, Nigeria. BMC Cancer. 2006; 26; 6:271.

8. Isara AR, Ojedokun CI. Knowledge of breast cancer and practice of breast self-examination among female senior secondary school students in Abuja, Nigeria. J Prev Med Hyg. 2011;52(4):186-190.

9. Pengpid S, Peltzer K. Knowledge, attitude and practice of breast self-examination among female university students from 24 low, middle income and emerging economy countries. Asian Pac J Cancer Prev. 2014; 15(20):8637-8640.

10. Olajide TO, Ugburo AO, Habeebu MO, Lawal AO, Afolayan MO, Mofikoya MO. Awareness and practice of breast screening and its impact on early detection and presentation among breast cancer patients attending a clinic in Lagos, Nigeria. Niger J Clin Pract. 2014;17(6):802-807.

11. Gwarzo UM, Sabitu K, Idris SH. Knowledge and practice of breast-self-examination among female undergraduate students of Ahmadu Bello University Zaria, northwestern Nigeria. Ann Afr Med. 2009;8(1):55-58.

12. Obajimi MO, Ajayi IO, Oluwasola AO, Adedokun BO, Adeniji-Sofoluwe AT, Mosuro OA, Akingbola TS, Bassey OS, Umeh E,

Soyemi TO, Adegoke F, Ogungbade I, Ukaigwe C, Olopade OI. Level of awareness of mammography among women attending outpatient clinics in a teaching hospital in Ibadan, South-West Nigeria. BMC Public Health. 2013; 16:13:40.

13. Sheppard VB, Christopher J, Nwabukwu I. Breaking the silence barrier: opportunities to address breast cancer in African-born women. J Natl Med Assoc. 2010;102(6):461-468.

14. Oguntola AS, Olaitan PB, Omotoso O, Oseni GO. Knowledge, attitude and practice of prophylactic mastectomy among patients and relations attending a surgical outpatient clinic. Pan Afr Med J. 2012; 13:20.

Chapter 16

Lack of access to diagnostic test to determine predisposition to Breast Cancer

In the developed world, there is a paradigm shift from treating diseases to managing predisposition to diseases. Nigeria and other developing countries will need to urgently learn from this evidenced based best practice. This will allow prophylactic remedies such as preventive surgery to be applied and thus free up resources that would have been required for the long term management of diseases. This can potentially improve the quality of life and reduce mortality for women with BRCA cancer genes. Women who carry the BRCA1 or BRCA2 cancer genes can reduce their risk of death, breast and ovarian cancer by getting preventive surgery. Women in developing countries should be able to make the choice to reduce their risk for breast cancer by getting tested for the BRCA mutations. If BRCA is positive, they must be able to decide like their counterparts in the developed world to undergo risk reducing prophylactic surgery to remove their breast. At the moment women in developing world do not enjoy this privilege. Women with high risk factors for breast cancer should be prime candidate for the BRCA gene test. *BRCA1* and *BRCA2* are the most common cause of hereditary breast cancer. In normal cells, these genes help prevent cancer by making proteins that keep the cells from growing abnormally. If you have inherited a mutated copy of either gene from a parent, you have a high risk of developing breast cancer during your lifetime. Although in some families with *BRCA1* mutations, the lifetime risk of breast cancer is as high as 80%; on average this risk seems to be in the range of 55% to 65%. For *BRCA2* mutations the risk is lower, around 45%. Women who have inherited mutations in the *BRCA1* or *BRCA2* (*BRCA1/2*) genes have substantially elevated risks of breast cancer and ovarian cancer, with a lifetime risk of breast cancer of 56% to 84%.[1-5] The estimated ovarian cancer risks range from 36% to 63% for *BRCA1* mutation carriers and 10% to 27% for *BRCA2* mutation carriers. Women who are mutation carriers have cancer risk management options that include risk reducing salpingo-oophorectomy, risk-reducing mastectomy, annual cancer screening, and chemoprevention. Due to the lack of effective screening for ovarian cancer, salpingo-oophorectomy is strongly recommended once childbearing is complete. In a prospective, multicentre cohort study of 2,482 women with *BRCA1* or *BRCA2* mutations ascertained between 1974 and 2008, no breast cancers were diagnosed in the 247 women with risk reducing mastectomy, compared with 98 women of 1372 diagnosed with breast cancer who did not have risk reducing mastectomy.[6] Women who are mutation carriers have cancer risk management options that include risk reducing mastectomy, annual cancer screening, and chemoprevention. Breast cancers linked to these mutations occur more often in younger women and more often affect both breasts than cancers not linked to these mutations. Women with these inherited mutations also have an increased risk for developing other cancers. In the United States, *BRCA* mutations are more common in Jewish people of Ashkenazi (Eastern Europe) origin than in other racial and ethnic groups, but they can occur in anyone. Other gene mutations can also lead to inherited breast cancers. These gene mutations are much rarer and often do not increase the risk of breast cancer as much as the *BRCA* genes.

The *ATM* gene is located at 11q22.3 and consists of 66 exons, 62 of which encode a protein of 3056 amino acids.[7] ATM belongs to a protein family known as the PI3K related protein kinases (PIKK). These proteins are characterized by a domain similar to that in phosphatidylinositol 3-kinase and most PIKKs, including ATM, are active serine/threonine kinases. ATM also contains a C-terminal FAT domain (*F*RAP, *A*TM, *T*RAPP), with a highly conserved 35 residue tail known as the FATC domain.[8] This domain appears to be important for regulating the kinase activity of ATM and for binding regulatory proteins.[9] Swift first proposed that relatives of ataxia-telangiectasia might be at increased risk of breast cancer nearly twenty years ago.[10] His analysis of cancer incidence in 110 ataxia-telangiectasia families suggested that the relative risk of cancer was 2.3 for men and 3.1 for women, with breast cancer being the most strongly associated cancer. The *ATM* gene normally helps repair damaged DNA. Inheriting 2 abnormal copies of this gene causes the disease ataxia-telangiectasia. Inheriting 1 mutated copy of this gene has been linked to a high rate of breast cancer in some families.

The *TP53* gene gives instructions for making a protein called p53 that helps stop the growth of abnormal cells. Inherited mutations of this gene cause *Li-Fraumeni syndrome* (named after the 2 researchers who first described it). People with this syndrome have an increased risk of developing breast cancer. TP53 are also key prognostic markers in breast cancer treatment.[11] TP53 mutation status and gene expression based groups are important survival markers of breast cancer, and these molecular markers may provide prognostic information that complements clinical variables. The study adds experience and knowledge to an ongoing characterization and classification of the disease.[12-13]

Mutations in the CHEK2 gene confer a moderately increased breast cancer risk. The risk for female carriers of the CHEK2*1100delC mutation is twofold increased. The Li-Fraumeni syndrome can also be caused by inherited mutations in the CHEK2 gene. Even when it does not cause this syndrome, it can increase breast cancer risk about twofold when it is mutated. In the general population, the CHEK2*1100delC mutation confers a slightly increased breast cancer risk, but in a familial breast cancer setting this risk is between 35%-55% for first degree female carriers. Female breast cancer patients with the CHEK2*1100delC mutation are at increased risk of contralateral breast cancer and may have a less favourable prognosis. Female heterozygous for CHEK2*1100delC mutation carriers are offered annual mammography and specialist breast surveillance between the ages of 35-60 years.[14]

There is need for diagnostic testing for biallelic mutations in CHEK2 in non BRCA1/2 breast cancer families, especially in populations with a relatively high prevalence of deleterious mutations in CHEK2.[15-17]

PTEN: The PTEN gene normally helps regulate cell growth. Inherited mutations in this gene can cause Cowden syndrome, a rare disorder in which people are at increased risk for both benign and malignant breast tumors, as well as growths in the digestive tract, thyroid, uterus, and ovaries. Defects in this gene can also cause a different syndrome called Bannayan-Riley-Ruvalcaba syndrome that is not thought to be linked to breast cancer risk. Recently, the syndromes caused by PTEN have been combined into one called PTEN Tumor Hamartoma Syndrome.[18-20]

CDH1: Women with mutations in this gene also have an increased risk of invasive lobular breast cancer.[21-23]

STK11: Defects in this gene can lead to Peutz-Jeghers syndrome. People with this disorder develop pigmented spots on their lips and in their mouths, polyps in the urinary and gastrointestinal tracts, and have an increased risk of breast cancer.[24-26]

PALB2: The PALB2 gene makes a protein that interacts with the protein made by the BRCA2 gene. Defects (mutations) in this gene can lead to an increased risk of breast cancer.[27-29]

References

1. Chen S, Parmigiani G. Meta-analysis of *BRCA1* and *BRCA2* penetrance. *J Clin Oncol*. 2007; 25(11):1329-1333.

2. Familial Breast Cancer: Classification and Care of People at Risk of Familial Breast Cancer and Management of Breast Cancer and Related Risks in People with a Family History of Breast Cancer. *National Collaborating Centre for Cancer (UK)*. 2013.

3. *Friebel TM, Domchek SM, Rebbeck TR*. Modifiers of cancer risk in BRCA1 and BRCA2 mutation carriers: systematic review and meta-analysis. *J Natl Cancer Inst*. 2014; 106(6):dju091.

4. King MC, Marks JH, Mandell JB.New York Breast Cancer Study Group. Breast and ovarian cancer risks due to inherited mutations in *BRCA1* and *BRCA2*. *Science*. 2003; 302(5645):643-646.

5. Struewing JP, Hartge P, Wacholder S, et al. The risk of cancer associated with specific mutations of *BRCA1* and *BRCA2* among Ashkenazi Jews. *N Engl J Med*. 1997; 336(20):1401-1408.

6. Domchek SM, Friebel TM, Singer CF, Evans DG, Lynch HT, Isaacs C, Garber JE, Neuhausen SL, Matloff E, Eeles R, Pichert G, Van t'veer

L, Tung N, Weitzel JN, Couch FJ, Rubinstein WS, Ganz PA, Daly MB, Olopade OI, Tomlinson G, Schildkraut J, Blum JL, Rebbeck TR. Association of risk-reducing surgery in BRCA1 or BRCA2 mutation carriers with cancer risk and mortality. *JAMA.* 2010; 304(9):967-975.

7. Savitsky K, Bar-Shira A, Gilad S, Rotman G, Ziv Y, Vanagaite L et al. *Science 1995*; 268: 1749–1753.

8. Bosotti R, Isacchi A, Sonnhammer FL. *Trends Biochem Sci. 2000;* 25: 225–227.

9. Jiang X, Sun Y, Chen S, Roy K, Price BD. (2006). *J Biol Chem* 281: 15741–15746.

10. Swift M, Reitnauer PJ, Morrell D, Chase CL. *N Engl J Med 1987*; 316: 1289–1294.

11. Zghair AN, Sinha DK, Kassim A, Alfaham M, Sharma AK. Differential Gene Expression of BRCA1,ERBB2 and TP53 biomarkers between Human Breast Tissue and Peripheral Blood Samples of Breast Cancer. Anticancer Agents Med Chem. 2015 Aug 24.

12. Langerød A, Zhao H, Borgan Ø, Nesland JM, Bukholm IR, Ikdahl T, Kåresen R, Børresen-Dale AL, Jeffrey SS.TP53 mutation status and gene expression profiles are powerful prognostic markers of breast cancer. Breast Cancer Res. 2007; 9(3):R30.

13. Overgaard J, Yilmaz M, Guldberg P, Hansen LL, Alsner J.TP53 mutation is an independent prognostic marker for poor outcome in both node-negative and node-positive breast cancer. Acta Oncol. 2000; 39(3):327-33.

14. Adank MA, Hes FJ, van Zelst-Stams WA, van den Tol MP, Seynaeve C, Oosterwijk JC. (2015). CHEK2-mutation in Dutch breast cancer families: expanding genetic testing for breast cancer. Ned Tijdschr Geneeskd 2015; 159:A8910.

15. Adank MA, Jonker MA, Kluijt I, van Mil SE, Oldenburg RA, Mooi WJ, Hogervorst FB, van den Ouweland AM, Gille JJ, Schmidt MK, van der Vaart AW, Meijers-Heijboer H, Waisfisz Q. CHEK2*1100delC

homozygosity is associated with a high breast cancer risk in women. J Med Genet 2011 ;48(12):860-863.

16. Oldenburg RA, Kroeze-Jansema K, Kraan J, Morreau H, Klijn JG, Hoogerbrugge N, Ligtenberg MJ, van Asperen CJ, Vasen HF, Meijers C, Meijers-Heijboer H, de Bock TH, Cornelisse CJ, Devilee P. The CHEK2*1100delC variant acts as a breast cancer risk modifier in non-BRCA1/BRCA2 multiple-case families. Cancer Res. 2003; 63(23):8153-8157.

17. Johnson N, Fletcher O, Naceur-Lombardelli C, dos Santos Silva I, Ashworth A, Peto J.Interaction between CHEK2*1100delC and other low-penetrance breast-cancer susceptibility genes: a familial study. Lancet. 2005 Oct 29-Nov 4;366(9496):1554-1557.

18. Nandini Dey, Brandon Young, Mark Abramovitz, Mark Bouzyk, Benjamin Barwick, Pradip De, Brian Leyland-Jones. Differential Activation of Wnt-β-Catenin Pathway in Triple Negative Breast Cancer Increases MMP7 in a PTEN Dependent Manner. PLoS One. 2013; 8(10): e77425.

19. Tuomas Heikkinen, Dario Greco, Liisa M Pelttari, Johanna Tommiska, Pia Vahteristo, Päivi Heikkilä, Carl Blomqvist, Kristiina Aittomäki, Heli Nevanlinna. Variants on the promoter region of *PTEN* affect breast cancer progression and patient survival. Breast Cancer Res. 2011; 13(6): R130.

20. Katherine Stemke-Hale, Ana Maria Gonzalez-Angulo, Ana Lluch, Richard M. Neve, Wen-Lin Kuo, Michael Davies, Mark Carey, Zhi Hu, Yinghui Guan, Aysegul Sahin, W. Fraser Symmans, Lajos Pusztai, Laura K. Nolden, Hugo Horlings, Katrien Berns, Mien-Chie Hung, Marc J. van de Vijver, Vicente Valero, Joe W. Gray, René Bernards, Gordon B. Mills, Bryan T. Hennessy. An Integrative Genomic and Proteomic Analysis of PIK3CA, PTEN, and AKT Mutations in Breast Cancer. Cancer Res. 2008 August 1; 68(15): 6084–6091.

21. Rodrigo Goncalves, Wayne A Warner, Jingqin Luo, Matthew J Ellis. New concepts in breast cancer genomics and genetics Breast Cancer Res. 2014; 16(5): 460.

22. Petra van der Groep, Elsken van der Wall, Paul J. van Diest. Pathology of hereditary breast cancer Cell Oncol (Dordr) 2011 April; 34(2): 71–88.

23. Roisin Connolly, Vered Stearns. Epigenetics as a Therapeutic Target in Breast Cancer. J Mammary Gland Biol Neoplasia.. 2012; 17(3-4): 191–204.

24. Tim Ripperger, Dorothea Gadzicki, Alfons Meindl, Brigitte Schlegelberger. Breast cancer susceptibility: current knowledge and implications for genetic counselling. Eur J Hum Genet. 2009 June; 17(6): 722–731.

25. Natalia Bogdanova, Sonja Helbig, Thilo Dörk. Hereditary breast cancer: ever more pieces to the polygenic puzzle. Hered Cancer Clin Pract. 2013; 11(1): 12.

26. Tuya Pal, Susan T. Vadaparampil. Genetic Risk Assessments in Individuals at High Risk for Inherited Breast Cancer in the Breast Oncology Care Setting. Cancer Control. 2012 October; 19(4): 255–266.

27. Zhi L Teo, Daniel J Park, Elena Provenzano, Catherine A Chatfield, Fabrice A Odefrey, Tu Nguyen-Dumont, kConFab, James G Dowty, John L Hopper, Ingrid Winship, David E Goldgar, Melissa C Southey. Prevalence of *PALB2* mutations in Australasian multiple-case breast cancer families. Breast Cancer Res. 2013; 15(1): R17.

28. Christian Bowman-Colin, Bing Xia, Samuel Bunting, Christiaan Klijn, Rinske Drost, Peter Bouwman, Laura Fineman, Xixi Chen, Aedin C. Culhane, Hong Cai, Scott J. Rodig, Roderick T. Bronson, Jos Jonkers, Andre Nussenzweig, Chryssa Kanellopoulou, David M. Livingston. *Palb2* synergizes with *Trp53* to suppress mammary tumor formation in a model of inherited breast cancer. Proc Natl Acad Sci U S A. 2013 May 21; 110(21): 8632–8637.

29. Yonglan Zheng, Jing Zhang, Qun Niu, Dezheng Huo, Olufunmilayo I. Olopade. Novel germline *PALB2* truncating mutations in African-American breast cancer patients. Cancer. 2012 March 1; 118(5): 1362–1370.

Chapter 17

Poor access to Breast Cancer diagnostic services in rural settings

In developing countries, late stages at presentation and poor diagnostic and treatment capacities contribute to lower breast cancer survival rates than in high-income countries. [1] Poor health within countries and inequities between countries are largely caused by the unequal distribution of power, income, goods, and services resulting from a combination of poor social policies, unfair economic arrangements, bad politics and corruption. [2] It is the downstream effect of social factors (such as nutritious food, clean water, sanitation, shelter, health care, literacy and meaningful work) that act in synergistic ways with genetics to determine the life expectancy of a population. With respect to access and financing, the health care system itself is a social determinant of individual health, and currently only 5% of global spending on cancer is directed toward developing countries. [2] Cancers that affect primarily women are a special subset of health inequality, as many women in developing countries lack access to screening and treatment as a consequence of discriminatory beliefs and practices. [3] Although the position of women has improved substantially over the past century in many developing countries, progress has been uneven and multiple challenges remain. [4]

Women's low literacy level, cultural and religious factors, competing health needs, limited resources, poorly developed health care services and limited information on cancer prevention are contributory factors. Women in rural areas tend to be less literate, more economically disadvantaged and more prone to cultural and religious marginalization. Economically disadvantaged women may also give less attention to their breast symptoms and/or be unable to use preventive measures due to a historical focus on curative medicine rather than preventive care. [4] Moreover the histopathological services they require may not be available in general hospitals in rural areas where a significant number of Nigerian women live. Sometimes when available, they are often beyond the reach of a vast majority. In most rural communities in Nigeria, there is widespread lack of health care professionals skilled in the diagnosis of breast cancer as well as in the administration of chemotherapeutic agents. Also access to laboratories for blood count analyses and effective antiemetic treatments are often lacking. A dismal 80% of breast cancer patients in Nigeria present at an advanced stage, requiring mastectomy; the majority are either dead or lost to follow-up within a year. [5] Low-income areas, such as sub-Saharan Africa, have the highest mortality rate in ages 45 to 59 years, with devastating effects on family structure and income. [6] Women particularly those in rural communities may conceal their symptoms to protect the integrity of a family's marginal finances. [7] Explanations for delayed clinical presentation include lack of education and awareness, superstition, denial, and fears of diagnosis with consequent disfiguring surgery. In addition, the majority of women in the world do not have access to screening mammography. [8]

Several factors contribute to the lack effective breast cancer services in rural settings; poor infrastructural facilities, suboptimal number of trained laboratory scientist in the field of histopathology, histopathologist and physicians in women's health, failure in stewardship by government in ensuring equitable distribution of health facilities and services, low wages for healthcare workers and poor infrastructural facilities (electricity, pipe borne water, roads and recreational activities). These factors contribute to the lack of access to life-saving breast cancer-related services in rural settings particularly in Nigeria. Also in Nigeria and other developing countries, the number of research personnel and skilled scientists are in limited supply. An insignificant less than 1% of national budgets is spent on research, there are few and often poorly endowed doctor training programs and often there are 1 or fewer scientists per million persons. [9] There is also the challenge of brain drain of valuable skilled professionals from developing countries to resource-rich countries. [10] Often when health professionals have opportunities to train in cancer centers in developed countries to gain additional training, there is often misplaced priorities as they often learn new innovative medical and surgical technologies rather than more helpful scientific methodology and preventive measures particularly because these new innovative medical and surgical technologies may not be available for them to use on their return. Scientific methodology and preventive measures would be more relevant and applicable upon return to their home countries. [11] Also a significant number of these health professional do not return to their home countries after acquiring these useful knowledge that could potentially be used to optimize the breast cancer service delivery. There is need for the Nigerian government to implement strategies to improve patient access and compliance as well as access to health-care professionals and policy-maker awareness that breast cancer is a cost-effective, treatable disease if detected early and managed effectively. The major challenge particularly in rural settings in Nigeria is that there is very little community awareness that breast cancer is treatable, inadequate advanced histopathology services for diagnosis and staging, fragmented treatment options and poor access to the full range of systemic treatments.

Geographic barriers are especially important for women who live in rural areas in Nigeria. These women may be unable to obtain regular breast cancer screening because they do not have access to these services in their local general hospitals. [12] Many women particularly those in rural areas will have to travel for several hours to access these services in urban centres. The roads are often poorly managed coupled with cost of transportation. These challenges can have a negative impacts on the quality of life of these rural women and affect their attitude towards screening and receive treatment. [13]

Access to finances is higher among urban dwellers compared to those in rural communities. Women with poor socioeconomic status (SES) are more likely to be rural dwellers. Financial barriers limit the ability of women, especially rural women in the poorest SES group from utilizing screening and treatment services for early diagnosis and treatment of breast cancer. [14]. Interventions that will improve financial risk protection for rural women with breast cancer or at risk of breast cancer as well as the availability of breast cancer screening and treatment services in rural hospitals are needed to ensure equitable access to breast cancer care. There is also the need for these services to be offered at affordable cost to these rural women. Socioeconomic, sociodemographic and health-system related characteristics are barriers to accessing breast cancer screening and treatment in developing countries. [13, 15-16] These barriers are mostly due to lower income, lower educational attainment, lack of appropriate health information, inequitable distribution of breast cancer services, lack of universal access to affordable healthcare services and failure in stewardship by the Nigerian government and managers of the healthcare system. The United Nations Report indicates that poverty is still deepening in Nigeria, with over 71.5% of the people living on less than one United States of America dollar a day. [17]

In Nigeria, screening, diagnostic and clinical services for breast cancer are grossly inadequate and there is often a higher urban-rural bias in the distribution of breast cancer-related services. Only few centres particularly in rural settings have breast cancer screening services, a functional and equipped histopathology laboratory, qualified laboratory scientist, histopathologist, functioning radiotherapy equipment and radiological services. Often in centres where these services are available, they are often suboptimal and above the reach of a vast majority of rural women. [18-19] The reasons why most breast cancer patients in Nigeria present late for treatment is not far-fetched. Most of the financial costs associated with breast cancer are paid through out-of-pocket, which is still the major healthcare financing mechanism in Nigeria. The Nigerian government will have to rise to her responsibility and sort out healthcare challenges surrounding lack of awareness, accessibility and financial constraints. Nigeria is an oil rich nations and can afford to offer her citizens the best quality of breast cancer services and care like her other counterparts in the world. The health budget has quadrupled over the last decade, yet access to healthcare services particularly for cancer has not improved in a commensurate manner due to corruption in governance. [20] In Nigeria the minimum monthly wage remains an insignificant eighteen thousand naira (N18,0000). Rural dwellers constitute a significant proportion of Nigerian with the poorest SES group. These women are often on lower income, poorly educated and involved in menial occupation and can hardly afford health insurance. For most of these women, the direct and indirect costs of obtaining breast cancer-related care and service can account for a substantial proportion of total household income. [21] Access and cost of diagnostic and medical treatment are major financial barrier to the continued benefit from breast cancer screening and treatment services especially among women in the poorest and very poor SES groups. [22] These women are less likely to utilize screening services, are significantly more likely to be diagnosed with a later-stage of breast cancer and to die from the disease. [23]

Health outcomes are better in urban than in rural areas of developing countries. [24] There is rural-urban gap in the access to breast cancer screening and treatment. Understanding the nature and the causes of this rural-urban disparity is essential to enable the government target resources appropriately to improve the health indices of rural dwellers. The Nigerian government need to develop a program that objectively target rural-urban disparity in access to healthcare services. Culturally and socially relevant educational material must be provided particularly to rural women in developing countries. There is the urgent need to provide basic amenities aimed at improving the quality of lives of rural dwellers, provide better incentives for healthcare workers posted to hospitals in rural communities, establish and maintain cancer data registries as well as provide multidisciplinary centres of excellence with broad outreach programmes to provide community access to cancer diagnosis and treatment.

References

1. Anderson BO, Cazap E, El Saghir NS, Yip CH, Khaled HM, Otero IV, Adebamowo CA, Badwe RA, Harford JB. Lancet Oncol. 2011; 12(4):387-398.

2. Marmot M, Friel S, Bell R, et al. Commission on Social Determinants of Health. Closing the gap in a generation: health equity through action on the social determinants of health. Lancet. 2008;372:1661–1669.

3. Wakabi W. Research collaboration boosts women's health in Ethiopia. Lancet. 2008;372:1534.

4. Pinotti JA, Faúndes A. Obstetric and gynecological care for Third World women. Int J Gynaecol Obstet. 1984;22:449–455.

5. Anyanwu SN. Temporal trends in breast cancer presentation in the third world. J Exp Clin Cancer Res. 2008;27:17.

6. Igene H. Global health inequalities and breast cancer: an impending public health problem for developing countries. Breast J. 2008;14:428–434.

7. Reeler A, Qiao Y, Dare L, et al. Women's cancers in developing countries: from research to an integrated health systems approach. Asian Pac J Cancer Prev. 2009;10:519–526.

8. Smith RA, Caleffi M, Albert US, et al. Global Summit Early Detection and Access to Care Panel. Breast cancer in limited-resource countries: early detection and access to care. Breast J. 2006;12(1):S16–S20.

9. Mellstedt H. Cancer initiatives in developing countries. Ann Oncol. 2006;17(8):24–31.

10. Serour GI. Healthcare workers and the brain drain. Int J Gynaecol Obstet. 2009;106:175–178.

11. Tobias JS, Mittra I. Improving cancer care worldwide. Ann Oncol. 1993;4:283–287.

12. Wang F, McLafferty S, Escamilla V, Luo L. Late-Stage breast cancer diagnosis and health care access in Illinois. Prof Geogr 2008;60:54-69.

13. MacKinnon JA, Duncan RC, Huang Y, Lee DJ, Fleming LE, Voti L, *et al.* Detecting an association between socioeconomic status and late stage breast cancer using spatial analysis and area-based measures. Cancer Epidemiol Biomarkers Prev 2007;16:756-762.

14. Okoronkwo IL, Ejike-Okoye P, Chinweuba AU, Nwaneri AC. Financial barriers to utilization of screening and treatment services for breast cancer: an equity analysis in Nigeria. Niger J Clin Pract. 2015 Mar-Apr;18(2):287-291.

15. Park MJ, Park EC, Choi KS, Jun JK, Lee HY. Sociodemographic gradients in breast and cervical cancer screening in Korea: The Korean National Cancer Screening Survey (KNCSS) 2005-2009. BMC Cancer 2011;11:257.

16. Ward E, Jemal A, Cokkinides V, Singh GK, Cardinez C, Ghafoor A, et al. Cancer disparities by race/ethnicity and socioeconomic status. CA Cancer J Clin 2004;54:78-93.

17. Human Development Report Nigeria 2008-2009: Achieving growth with equity, Nigeria: UNDP. www.ng.undp.org/documents/NHDR2009.

18. Okobia MN, Bunker CH, Okonofua FE, Osime U. Knowledge, attitude and practice of Nigerian women towards breast cancer: A cross-sectional study. World J Surg Oncol 2006;4:11.

19. Onwere S, Okoro O, Chigbu B, Aluka C, Kamanu C, Onwere A. Breast self-examination as a method of early detection of breast cancer: Knowledge and practice among antenatal clinic attendees in South Eastern Nigeria. Pak J Med Sci 2009;25:122-125.

20. Onwujekwe O, Hanson K, Uzochukwu B. Examining inequities in incidence of catastrophic health expenditures on different healthcare services and health facilities in Nigeria. PLoS One 2012;7:e40811.

21. Ichoku HE, Fonta W. The distributive effect of health care financing in Nigeria. PEP Working Paper, No 2006-17. Canada: University of Laval. http://www.portal.pep-net.org/documents/download/id/13555.

22. Egwuonwu OA, Anyanwu SN, Nwofor AM. Default from neoadjuvant chemotherapy in premenopausal female breast cancer patients: What is to blame? Niger J Clin Pract 2012;15:265-269.

23. Schueler KM, Chu PW, Smith-Bindman R. Factors associated with mammography utilization: A systematic quantitative review of the literature. J Womens Health (Larchmt). 2008;17:1477-1498.

24. Van de Poel E, O'Donnell O, Van Doorslaer E. Are urban children really healthier? Evidence from 47 developing countries. Soc Sci Med. 2007 ;65(10):1986-2003.

Chapter 18

Pregnancy and breast cancer in Nigeria

Breast cancer in pregnancy accounts for 2%–3% of all breast cancers. The increased vascularity and lymphatic drainage from the breast during pregnancy potentiate the metastatic spread of the cancer to the regional lymph nodes. The detection rates of breast lesions by both CBE and breast ultrasonography were equivalent during pregnancy and 6 weeks postpartum, making CBE a convenient and very cost effective method of detecting breast lesions in the low risk population. However, both CBE and breast ultrasonography should be done in women with high risk of breast malignancy.[1] The frequency of pregnancy- associated breast cancer, a rare but serious occurrence, may increase in light of the secular trends for lower parity in general and for older age at first full-term delivery in particular. Women treated with fertility treatment drugs may be at a higher risk for Pregnancy Associated Breast Cancer (PABC).[2-4] Breast cancers appear to be associated with distinct reproductive risk factors, highlighting the need for better understanding of the biological bases of early BC in African populations.[5] Parity may have different roles in the development of PABC versus other premenopausal breast cancer in Nigerian women. Prospective mothers with multiple births and a family history of breast cancer may have an elevated risk of breast cancer during their immediate postpartum period.[6] Post-partum breast involution may be responsible for the increased metastatic potential of post-partum PABC.[7-8] Breast cancer is a leading cause of cancer morbidity and mortality for women worldwide.[9-10]

References

1. Ezeonu PO, Ajah LO, Onoh RC, Lawani LO, Enemuo VC, Agwu UM. Evaluation of clinical breast examination and breast ultrasonography

among pregnant women in Abakaliki, Nigeria. Onco Targets Ther. 2015 May 13;8:1025-9.

2. Bell RJ, Fradkin P, Parathithasan N, Robinson PJ, Schwarz M, Davis SR. Pregnancy-associated breast cancer and pregnancy following treatment for breast cancer, in a cohort of women from Victoria, Australia, with a first diagnosis of invasive breast cancer. Breast. 2013; 22(5):980-985.

3. Callihan EB, Gao D, Jindal S, Lyons TR, Manthey E, Edgerton S, Urquhart A, Schedin P, Borges VF. Postpartum diagnosis demonstrates a high risk for metastasis and merits an expanded definition of pregnancy-associated breast cancer. Breast Cancer Res Treat. 2013; 138(2):549-559.

4. Keinan-Boker L, Lerner-Geva L, Kaufman B, Meirow D.Pregnancy-associated breast cancer. Isr Med Assoc J. 2008;10(10):722-727.

5. Sighoko D, Kamaté B, Traore C, Mallé B, Coulibaly B, Karidiatou A, Diallo C, Bah E, McCormack V, Muwonge R, Bourgeois D, Gormally E, Curado MP, Bayo S, Hainaut P.Breast cancer in pre-menopausal women in West Africa: analysis of temporal trends and evaluation of risk factors associated with reproductive life. Breast. 2013; 22(5):828-835.

6. Hou N, Ogundiran T, Ojengbede O, Morhason-Bello I, Zheng Y, Fackenthal J, Adebamowo C, Anetor I, Akinleye S, Olopade OI, Huo D. Risk factors for pregnancy-associated breast cancer: a report from the Nigerian Breast Cancer Study. Ann Epidemiol. 2013; 23(9):551-557.

7. Lyons TR, Schedin PJ, Borges VF. Pregnancy and breast cancer: when they collide. J Mammary Gland Biol Neoplasia. 2009;14(2):87-98.

8. Kasum M, Beketić-Orešković L, Orešković S.Subsequent pregnancy and prognosis in breast cancer survivors. Acta Clin Croat. 2014; 53(3):334-341.

9. Anothaisintawee T, Wiratkapun C, Lerdsitthichai P, Kasamesup V, Wongwaisayawan S, et al. (2013) Risk factors of breast cancer: a systematic review and meta-analysis. Asia Pac J Public Health 25: 368–387.

10. Warner E. Clinical practice. Breast-cancer screening. N Engl J Med.2011; 365: 1025–1032.

Way Forward with Breast Cancer in Nigeria

Worldwide, breast cancer is the commonest cancer in women and it is characterized by regional variations and late clinical presentation in low and middle income countries including Nigeria. There is an urgent need to step up activities through governmental and non-governmental agencies to promote advocacy, national policy on training of personnel for diagnosis, clinical and self-breast examination and nationwide screening program (mammography), in order to enhance early detection, control the upward trends and reduce the mortality rate from breast cancer. Routine age appropriate and specific breast cancer screening should become an integral part of healthcare system in Nigeria allowing for early detection and intervention; aggressive awareness campaign on the advantages of early diagnosis and the dangers of late presentation, need to offer universal and affordable treatment, provision of health education, encouraging our women to conduct routine Breast Self Examination (BSE), implementation of a strategy to offer annual mammogram to women above the age threshold for breast cancer, increased budgetary allocation for the diagnosis and management of cancer, more investment in the training of healthcare workers involved in the diagnosis and management of breast cancer in Nigeria. There is need to re-emphasize the importance of prompt reporting of any new breast symptoms to a health professional. Clinical Breast Examination (CBE) must become part of a periodic health examination, preferably at least every three years. Asymptomatic women aged 40 and above should be offered a CBE as part of a periodic health examination, preferably annually. Annual mammography should also be made available from the age of 40 years.

INDEX

A

Abraxane 27
Abuja Population Based Cancer
    Registry 66
AC 27, 31, 33, 46, 56, 95, 122
Acute Myeloid Leukaemia 27
Adriamycin 27, 71
African American Women 34, 41, 46,
    93, 95, 107
American Society of Plastic
    Surgeons 22
Anaemia 27
Anthracyclines 27
Apocrine metaplasia 80
Aromatase Inhibitors 48
Ashkenazi Jews 113
AT viii, 1, 3, 4, 6, 9, 12, 14, 17, 18, 20,
    23, 24, 27, 30, 33, 35, 36, 38,
    41, 42, 44, 50, 57, 58, 61, 65,
    66, 70, 72, 74, 77, 80, 87, 88,
    92, 94, 97, 98, 101, 103, 105,
    106, 108, 110, 112, 116, 118,
    121, 124, 127
Ataxia-telangiectasia 111, 112
ATM Gene 111
Atypia 39, 79
Atypical ductal hyperplasia 79
Atypical lobular hyperplasia 79

B

Biopsy 18, 31, 33, 67
Body Mass Index 53, 72, 78, 83
BRCA1 32, 36, 50, 82, 110, 112, 114
BRCA2 32, 36, 82, 98, 110, 113, 114
Breast Cancer Surgery 14, 60
Breast Lump 14, 45, 97, 106
Breast Self-Examination 34, 87, 89,
    90, 107, 108, 123

C

Capecitabine 27
Carboplatin 27
Cardiomyopathy 27
CDH1 113
CHEK2 83, 112, 114
Chemotherapy 5, 12, 20, 25, 26, 28,
    29, 32, 34, 39, 49, 59, 60, 68,
    71, 75, 95, 98, 107, 123
Cisplatin 27
Clinical Breast Examination vii, 31,
    32, 34, 86, 88, 106, 124, 127
CMF 27
CXCR4 52, 56
Cyclophosphamide 27, 71
Cytoxan 27

D

Diethylstilbestrol 79
Docetaxel 27

Doxil 27
Doxorubicin 27

E

Ellence 27
Epirubicin 27
Eribulin 27
ER Modulators 48
European Cancer Observatory 17

F

FAC 27
Familial Breast Cancer 21, 36, 78, 112
Fibroadenoma 68, 79
Fibrosarcoma 97
Fine Needle Aspiration 33
Flow Cytometry 67
Fluorouracil 27

G

Gemcitabine 27
Gemzar 27
Gynecomastia 99

H

Halaven 27
Hamartoma 80, 113
Hemangioma 80
HER2 27, 39, 48, 50, 52
Herceptin 27, 71
Hormone Replacement Therapy 2, 73
Hospital Based Cancer Registry 3

I

Ibadan Population Based Cancer Registry 66
Image Guided Radiotherapy 26
Immunotherapy 12

Infiltrating Ductal Carcinoma 14
Intensity Modulated Radiotherapy 26
International Agency for Research on Cancer 7, 40, 71
Intraoperative Radiation 26, 28
Invasive Ductal Carcinoma 15, 49, 97
Ixabepilone 27
Ixempra 27

K

Ketorolac 59, 60, 63, 64

L

Leucopenia 27
Leukaemia 27
Li-fraumeni syndrome 112
Lipoma 80
Liposomal 27
Lumina A 51
Lumina B 51
Lumpectomy 12, 25, 71

M

Magnetic Resonance Imaging 32, 35, 36
Male Breast Cancer 20, 67, 97, 98, 100, 102, 104
Mammogram vii, 17, 18, 20, 23, 31, 32, 36, 72, 79, 127
Mastectomy 12, 14, 16, 25, 26, 60, 63, 68, 71, 93, 94, 98, 103, 107, 109, 111, 118
Mastopexy 17
MDM2 50
Menopausal 6, 13, 39, 40, 78, 86, 125
Metabolic Equivalent of Task 78
Metaplastic Breast Cancer 14, 16
Methotrexate 27

Mitoxantrone 27
Modified radical mastectomy 13, 15, 98
Myelodysplastic Syndrome 27

N

Nab-paclitaxel 27
National Health Insurance Scheme 66
Navelbine 27
Neoadjuvant Chemotherapy 26, 28, 32, 34, 123
Neurofibroma 80
Neutrophil/Lymphocyte ratio 60
NICE 21, 32, 36
Nigeria v, vii, viii, ix, 1, 2, 4, 5, 6, 7, 8, 9, 10, 11, 13, 14, 15, 16, 17, 19, 20, 21, 23, 24, 26, 27, 28, 29, 30, 31, 32, 33, 34, 38, 39, 40, 41, 42, 44, 45, 46, 47, 48, 49, 50, 51, 54, 55, 57, 58, 59, 61, 65, 66, 67, 68, 69, 70, 71, 72, 73, 74, 75, 76, 77, 78, 80, 81, 84, 85, 86, 87, 89, 90, 91, 92, 93, 94, 95, 96, 98, 99, 100, 101, 102, 103, 105, 106, 107, 108, 109, 110, 118, 119, 120, 122, 123, 124, 125, 127
Non-Steroidal Anti-Inflammatory Drug 24, 59, 63
NSAID 21, 59, 60, 64
Nuclear Atypia 39

O

Obesity 4, 53, 77, 79, 80, 82, 83
Oestrogen Receptors 49

P

P21 50
P53 49, 50, 54, 55, 98, 112
Paclitaxel 27
PALB2 113, 116
Pancytopenia 27
Papillomatosis 79
P-cadherin 50
Periductal fibrosis 80
Perjeta 27
Pertuzumab 27
Peutz-Jeghers Syndrome 113
PgR 49, 50
PI3K 111
Pleomorphism 39
Pregnancy Associated Breast Cancer 124
Premenopausal 15, 29, 31, 34, 38, 46, 50, 67, 77, 78, 80, 84, 86, 123, 124
Progesterone Receptors 49, 52, 53, 54, 64

R

Radionuclide 39
Radiotherapy 14, 16, 20, 25, 26, 28, 45, 59, 66, 68, 71, 120
Randomized Clinical Trial 57, 58, 59, 62

S

Scirrhous 67
Scleroderma 25
Sclerosing Adenosis 79, 80
Stereotactic Body Radiotherapy 26
Supraclavicular lymphadenopathy 89

T

Tamoxifen 71, 98, 99, 103
Taxanes 27

Taxol 27
Taxotere 27
Thrombocytopenia 27
TP53 78, 83, 112, 114
Trastuzumab 27, 39
Triple Negative Breast Cancer vii, 48, 49, 50, 51, 55, 56, 58, 60, 67, 115
Tumours 13, 14, 15, 25, 48, 49, 50

U

Ultrasonography 32, 34, 86, 89, 124, 125
Union for International Cancer Control 71

V

Vinorelbine 27
Volumetric Arc Therapy 26

X

Xeloda 27

www.ingramcontent.com/pod-product-compliance
Lightning Source LLC
Chambersburg PA
CBHW030758180526
45163CB00003B/1073